# Yoga Without Boundaries

*By*

*Vani Devi*

The writer/publisher of this book does not accept responsibility for any accident, injury or problem caused by practising the breath work, meditations or postures in this book. Not all postures and practices are appropriate for all people. It is your responsibility to know your body and its limitations and to choose suitable practices. Please read the 'Cautions and Health Issues' before commencing your practice and consult a medical practitioner if necessary.

Published by Kool Kat Publications, 1 Dene Way, Newbury, Berks, RG14 2JL

Tel: 00 44 (0)1635 45300
E-mail: koolkatpub@hotmail.com
www.koolkatpublications.co.uk.

# Contents

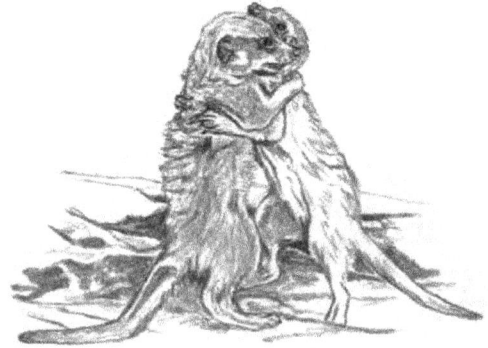

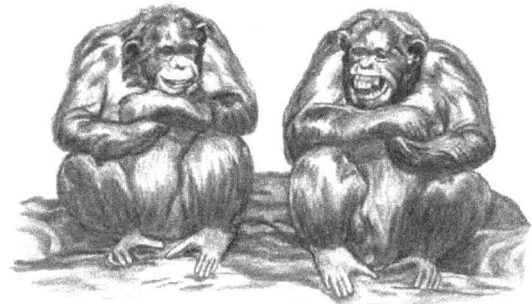

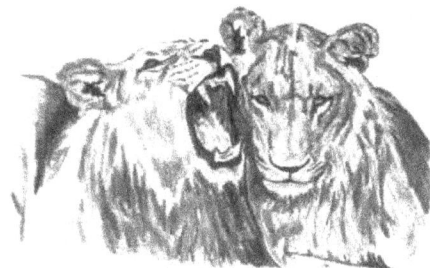

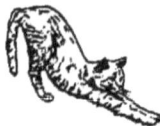

# Preface

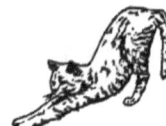

The title of this book, **Yoga without Boundaries**, is rather obscure. It may seem strange to some people. It is influenced by my love of **Vedanta** philosophy. Rather than expand about that here, I will use the spaces in the pages at the end of sections to explain it and delve into the concept of Vedanta, see pages **48**, **63**, **73** and **93**.

## The style of the book

I taught children the guitar in schools until I was 72 and still work, part-time, in a care home for adults with special needs. I keep these groups of clientele in mind when I write my books. I am more artistic than academic and the more I learn, the more humble I feel. I continue to write books because I get positive feedback and I feel the need to consolidate the many inspiring yogic ideas being manifested at this explosive time in the history of humanity. I prefer books to computer screens, although the internet has been a boon for spiritual practice and I frequently use it to source information and ideas.

I have kept the language of this book simple because yoga is for everybody and long words and too many intellectual demands can create a negative response. For this reason, I have not used many Sanskrit words, although I love this ancient Indian language.

Readers tell me they like the animal pictures. They offer light relief and celebrate nature and the wonders of Creation.

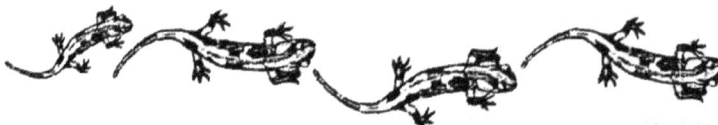

## The Content

I have named the sources of ideas whenever possible. With the exception of a few postures from the Supple Body Sequence all are from Yoga or Chi Gong backgrounds.

Essential content from my previous Yoga books is included in pages **6 - 15, 18 - 19, 23** and **74**. The **Full Yogic Breath** is a prerequisite for all yoga practices and an understanding of the **Sympathetic and Parasympathetic Nervous Systems** helps all areas of life. There can be no true involvement with Yoga until the basic awareness of the breath is appreciated.

As I teach mixed ability classes, it is necessary to develop different ways of practising the postures. Also, as yoga teaching in most countries is usually taught in weekly classes, the class routine becomes part of pupil's lives. I have met teachers who have been teaching the same pupils on this basis for up to 40 years. Although repetition is an essential part of yoga practice, innovation is necessary to keep the lessons interesting and develop potential.

People ask me if the illustrations are drawings or photographs. They are both. I take photos of my pupils, trace the outlines, fill in the details and then add the copied heads. You can tell which sections I completed in the 2020 Corona Virus lockdowns because my lodger Fabio and I are modelling the sequences.

## Acknowledgements

I would like to thank all my pupils for their encouragement and participation in my classes. They are my guinea pigs, the ones I use to try out new ideas and without them my books would not have been written.

I would like to thank Walter Krasniqi and Helen Cooper from Savvy Book Marketing, for supervising the production of this book. Also, my proof-reader, Rachel Tapping, and Elisa Burato, M.Ost., Bob Camp, Tasha Walker and Robert Moses for their contributions. Finally, my thanks go to Griff Johnson for his patience and expertise, when helping me produce the CD/Audio Track that can be used with this book.

## My background information

I studied guitar and singing at the Guildhall School of music in the 1960s. Kate Oppel (nee Stuckey) is my married name.  My first career was teaching the guitar in schools and as a singer guitarist at various events.  In my early forties, I had a consultation with a Harley Street speech therapist about a problem that developed at the age of ten.  The therapist advised me, 'I can't do anything for you but I suggest you take up Yoga'.  About two years later I finally made it to a local class and yoga has subsequently become an essential part of my life.

I took the Sivananda Yoga Teachers Training Course in the Bahamas in 1998.  I was given my spiritual name there.  **Vani Devi** means **Goddess of Speech and Song**.  I started teaching straight away in local village halls and the Pinnacle Leisure Centre (now Nuffield Health) in Newbury.  In 2001, I started teaching people in Reading whose lives had been disrupted by mental health issues. In the same year, I took the Sivananda Advanced Course in Canada.  I have taught young offenders in Reading Prison and patients in the psychiatric hospital in Reading and am still teaching mentally and physically vulnerable people.

In 2004, I took a Sivananda Sadhana Intensive in the Himalayas and again in France in 2005 and 2007.  The course involves studying the *Hatha Yoga Pradipika*, see **Glossary,** and going deeper into the practice of **Pranayama** (exploring the potential of the breath).  I feel it is the energy I generated during these courses that facilitated my book writing.  I took another similar **Hatha Intensive** in the Himalayas with Sivananda Yoga Vidya Peetham in 2018. That is where I was taught by Robert Moses who contributed the **Warm Up** section.

Meanwhile, I am very fortunate to live in an area that is overflowing with yogic activity. There are frequent workshops where all the different schools of yoga can be explored. British Wheel of Yoga Congresses and the World Yoga Festivals held in Pangbourne, Berkshire, have also been catalytic.

**Books self-published by the Author**
*Blues Guitar, Play it your Way* (Kate Oppel), 1994
*Yoga Sequences* (2003)
*Yoga Sequences Book 2* (2007)
*Yoga Expanded and Simplified* (2009)
*Yoga Sequences Companion*:  A compilation of
previous publications and new material. (2011)
*Yoga Footsteps* (2017)

**Published by Yoga Words**, an imprint of Pinter and Martin Ltd. London, SW2 1PS
**2nd Edition of *Yoga Sequences Companion*** (2015)
**Reprint** (2017)

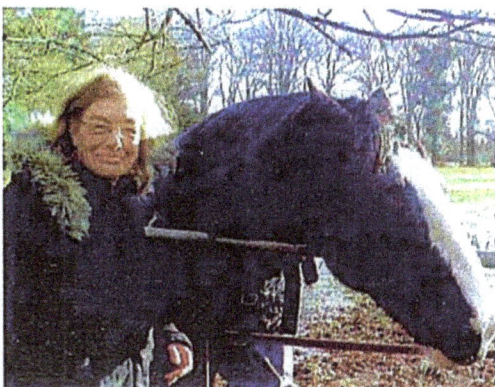

## Salutations from the Author

*May your yoga bring you joy and contentment.*

*Love and Light and rivers of OM*
*from*

Vani Devi

# Foreword

**Yoga Without Boundaries** truly makes yoga accessible to everyone and will offer new insight and practices to even the most learned teacher or student. I have been teaching yoga for 21 years and was thrilled to find a host of new ideas and techniques that could be used in my yoga therapy work and taught to my trainee yoga therapists at the Minded Institute.

Via its gently spoken and poetic narrative, Vani Devi takes the reader on a journey of yoga sequences she has learned or developed through the years. The landscape she creates allows us to view the many different yoga leaders and teachers that have contributed to an array of modern yoga and additional mind-body practices, revealing the organic evolution of modern-day yoga. Her own modifications and innovations remind us all that authentic yoga teaching is not a stagnant group of practices, but an emergence where ancient wisdom meets the reality of another person's body in the present moment, and responds with kindness and knowing.

Adding to this implicit but strongly felt reminder, her descriptions are light and clear and help, lull the reader into a yogic mindset necessary to begin practice. Truly the artist, with her own drawing peppered beautifully throughout the text, Vani Devi knows how to craft the journey to a yogic path for anyone, no matter their belief, needs, age or previous experience. I found myself entering a semi-meditative state in simply reading it. From simple mudra movements with the hands, that can be done by anyone, to the therapeutic yoga sequences for sciatica, to a gamut of meditations that can help quell a multitude of minds, Vani reveals her skills as a yoga teacher.

**Heather Mason**, founder of **The Minded Institute**.

www.themindedinstitute.com

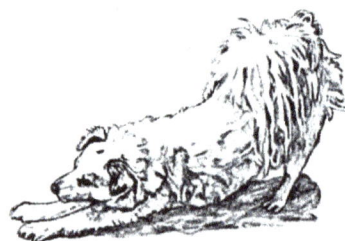

## The Basic Framework of Yoga

### The Four Paths of Yoga

**Lord Krishna**, who lived about 2,000BC, spoke about these four paths. His teachings were transmitted aurally for many generations and finally narrated in the **Bhagavad Gita** (c.600-500BC).

**Karma Yoga, the Yoga of action.** This is selfless service towards our fellow human beings, the Planet Earth and the Higher Consciousness with no thought of personal reward. Deeds, not words are important. The good and bad usage of words corresponds to deeds.

**Bhakti Yoga, the Yoga of Devotion.** This is an emotional longing for involvement with the cosmos and Higher Consciousness. Words are not used to justify the emotion but to express it in singing and chanting, ceremony, ritual and story telling.

**Raja Yoga, the Yoga of Meditation.** This is mind control with the goal of achieving higher states of consciousness. The asanas and contents of this book belong to this path. The body is controlled as a prelude to controlling the mind. Particular attention is paid to the movement of prana (life force) in the body. This is **Hatha Yoga**. The asana is one of several techniques used for controlling the life force in Hatha Yoga. In Raja Yoga words become superfluous; 'I don't think, therefore I am'.

**Jana Yoga, the Yoga of Knowledge.** It uses the intellect to ask questions, read, reflect and analyse. It transcends the unreal and negates bondage to the material world. It is dependent on words until the mind transcends the intellect.

All paths lead to the union of the individual self with the universal self. You are advised to follow the path that suits your personality but to practise all the other paths to some degree. The usage of words is my own suggestion, to simplify the understanding.

As we hold the postures in a state of bodily concentration and words become superfluous, we may, without realising it, experience this union, if only for a split second. The same applies during the usual final relaxation in a yoga class, and when we meditate.

## The Eight Limbs of Raja Yoga

**Patanjali** is thought to have lived between 2nd century BC and 4th century AD. 2,000 years ago there were many different schools of yoga. He attempted to clarify and consolidate them in his Yoga Sutras.

It is the practical content of the **Patanjali Sutras** that has received the most recognition. This includes **The Eight Limbs of Raja Yoga.** Some would consider this the 'back bone' of yoga.

# Limbs, steps or stages of Raja Yoga

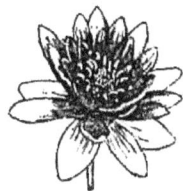

**1. Yama**, social conduct. **2. Niyama**, personal conduct. **3. Asanas**, postures.

**4. Pranayama**, control of prana, life force, cosmic energy through breathing.

**5. Pratyahara**, withdrawal of the senses.

6. **Dharana**, concentration. **7. Dhyana**, meditation. **8. Samadhi**, the bliss or super-conscious state.

# Cautions and Health Issues

People can hurt themselves putting out the garbage, turning over in bed and bending down to pick up something. It is obvious that care must be taken when practising yoga postures. As physical activities go, yoga has a good track record, although one hears of the occasional trapped nerve or accident. Dancers are much more likely to hurt themselves and athletes and football players have a shorter than average life expectancy.

Most of the feedback I have received about my books has been from yoga teachers. A few people told me they practised from them at home and didn't attend a class. These are the ones that need extra guidance and I am writing here with them in mind.

I prefer to distinguish between the fit and unfit, the well-coordinated and the uncoordinated, rather than the beginner and non-beginner. Some people do demanding postures with complete composure and confidence in their first yoga class. Some are used to listening to their bodies: others have lost touch with their bodies and need to develop this skill. Patience is also needed. It is important not to try too hard. Always keep within your comfort zone.

Wait until your body has warmed up before practising demanding stretches and twists. You are less likely to hurt yourself if you coordinate your breath with your posture work. Always connect to the breath. Stop if there is any discomfort. Don't hold the postures for too long at first. Move slowly and carefully from one posture to another.

## Here are some recognised precautions

If you have a particular physical problem, consult a medical practitioner before starting your practice. Advice varies; if in doubt, seek a second opinion.

If you have **high blood pressure**, it is advisable not to lower your head below the heart, unless you are used to doing this with no ill effects. Care is also needed in inverted postures[1], e.g. the **Head Stand** and **Shoulder Stand**. Taking the hips above the head may not be advisable, although some people with high blood pressure are quite comfortable in inverted postures. Some experimentation is necessary.

**Pregnant** women should lie on their left-hand side during relaxation. Also, they should not put pressure on the abdomen by lying face downwards.

If you have a **heart problem** or are **pregnant**, don't hold your breath for more than about ten seconds.

Avoid inverted postures if you suffer from **glaucoma, detached retina, neck problems** or have an **ear infection**. Some **pregnant** women are fine doing them: others may faint or have difficulty, so proceed with great caution.

When you are inverted, do not turn your head from side to side. Always look upwards.

**Neck** and **back problems** vary greatly. Find out which postures help your condition and avoid those that don't. Your medical practitioner should be able to advise you if necessary.

If you have taken **pain killers**, take care not to over-stretch during your posture work as signals to the brain will be suppressed.

1. The only inverted postures in this book are in the **Piriformis Stretch Sequence** on page 79.

# The Full Yogic Breath

**I CONSIDER** the **Full Yogic Breath** to be one of the most important things I have learnt in my life. Unfortunately I was not taught it until I did my Yoga Teachers Training Course. Meditation comes close behind in order of importance, because good breathing is a prerequisite to good meditation. High upper chest breathing, with lack of harmony between the diaphragm and the abdomen, will limit the development of your meditation.

## Method

1. Lie on your back. The legs can be straight or slightly bent. Place your hands on the lower abdomen. Breathe with a completely relaxed abdomen. You will feel the abdomen rise on the inhalation, under the influence of the diaphragm, and flatten on the exhalation as the diaphragm contracts up into the rib cage. **Diaphragmatic breathing** brings air into the bottom part of your lungs.

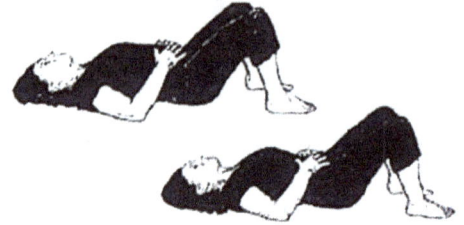

2. Keep the left hand on the abdomen and place your right hand on the diaphragm. Direct your breath to the bottom of your lungs. Feel both hands rising and falling with the breath. *Repeat three times.*

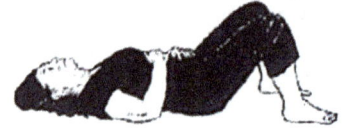

3. Place your right hand half way up the right side of the rib cage. The thumb should be at the back and your fingers wrapped around the front of your ribs. INHALE into the middle part of your lungs. The ribs should move up and out to the sides on the inhalation, and lower on the exhalation. The abdomen will also rise and fall with the breath. *Repeat three times.*

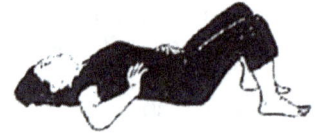

4. Place your right hand on the upper chest and INHALE into the top part of the lungs. The right hand will rise as the sternum, ribs and area below the neck (the clavicles) lift up and out. The left hand on the abdomen will not rise. *Repeat three times.*

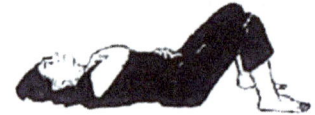

5. Now use all areas of the lungs; bottom, middle and top. This is the **Full Yogic Breath**. As you INHALE, fill the lungs from the bottom upwards, as if you were filling a glass of water. Both hands will rise. EXHALE from the top to the bottom, as if you were emptying a glass of water. Both hands will lower. *Repeat three times.*

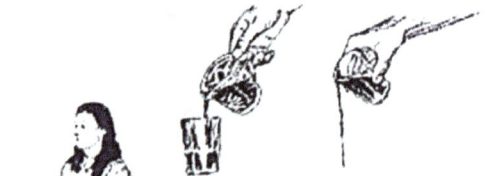

6. Sit in **Easy Pose** with the legs lightly crossed, or in another comfortable sitting position. Interlock the fingers in **Venus Lock**. Lower your hands with the palms facing downwards. EXHALE completely and then INHALE into the bottom part of the lungs. Feel everything around the waist expand.

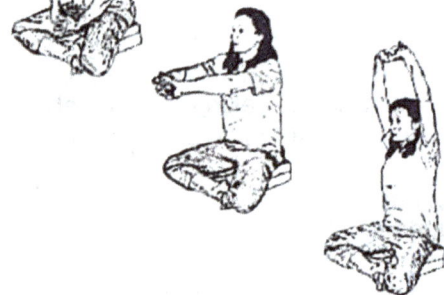

7. Continue to INHALE as you bring your arms up parallel to the floor, and breathe into the middle part of the lungs. Feel the ribs move up and out.

8. Raise your hands above your head and fill the top part of your lungs. Push away with the palms of your hands. This lifts the rib cage even further. Hold briefly.

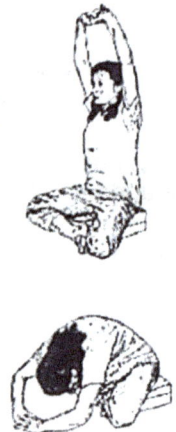

9. To EXHALE reverse the procedure. Lower your hands slowly as you empty the lungs from top, middle to bottom. To completely empty the bottom part of the lungs, soften the elbows and lean forward and down. Use the abdominal muscles to squeeze the last bit of air out. INHALE the head up. Repeat from **6** to **9** three times.

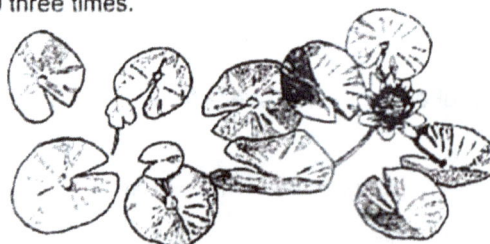

# Breathing

**The breath** is very important in yogic thinking. When we inhale, we not only take in oxygen, we take in **prana** (life force or cosmic energy) and breathing is our link to the cosmos. When we inhale, we think of building up a store of energy in the abdomen. It is psychologically healthy to be aware of this grounding, calming and strengthening force in the abdomen.

Traditionally, the yogic inhalation has been with a relaxed abdomen. This is how animals and babies breathe when they are relaxed. When they are active and agitated, the activity can move higher up into the lungs. When you breathe, your whole trunk from the top of your thighs to half way up the neck should move. Scientists have picked up minute movements in the bones of the skull during the breathing process.

As the diaphragm flattens and extends, everything around the waist should move. When I was studying singing at the Guildhall School of Music in the 60s, I was taught to expand around the waist when I breathed in. The abdominal muscles engage automatically on the exhalation to support the outgoing breath. I had the good fortune to come across a copy of **The Week** magazine in my dentist's waiting room. It contained an article about Tanya Streeter who held the record for deep sea diving at that time. She could hold her breath for 6 minutes and 17 seconds. She said that when she got ready to dive, she breathed in so much air that her stomach swelled up until it looked as if she was six months pregnant. We need not go to such extremes!

In Pilates, a slight contraction of the abdomen is recommended on the inhalation. This is understandable as Pilates was created with the ballet dancer in mind. An expanded abdomen would spoil the body line for dancing. Also, the abdominal muscles support the spine during movement. I went to one yoga class where the teacher taught Pilates breathing and decided it was definitely not for me, but yoga can accommodate differences of opinion.

Practising yoga makes you aware of your breathing and the potential expansion of the rib cage. Many people breathe in an unhealthy way for most of their lives. Yoga can correct this. You are never too old to take up yoga. When I took my Yoga Teachers Training Course, I wasn't particularly flexible. By the time I reached my 60s, I was much more flexible and I had more energy. More importantly, I became a more compassionate, aware human being. Interestingly, the very talented horoscope writer, the late Jonathan Cainer, wrote just before I took my Yoga TTC, 'You are about to start a new career and it is going to be very good for your social life'. That has proved to be very accurate. Yet another perk that comes with the yoga journey.

Most people breathe between fifteen and twenty times a minute. The breath is closely linked to mental activity. When we are agitated, we breathe quickly. When we listen acutely, we stop breathing. When we slow down our breathing, we become calm.

## Experimenting with breath and emotions

To experience this connection, experiment with feeling different emotions. Observe the speed of your breathing and which parts of the body are moving. Here are some suggestions:

*Imagine you are relaxing in a hot bath*

*Feel very angry*

*You are warm and cosy in bed and about to fall asleep*

*Feel very frightened*

*Imagine you are stroking an animal you love very much*

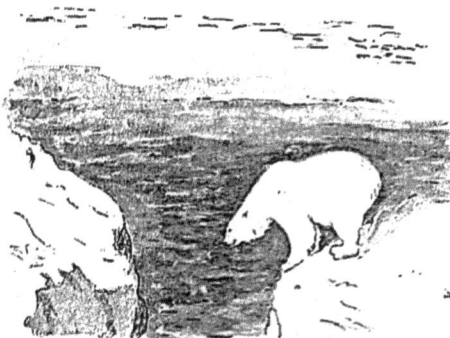

*Imagine you are an actor or musician about to perform a demanding part*

*Feel very happy*

*Feel very sad*

*Imagine you are about to meet somebody who is important to you. You haven't seen them for a long time and you are both excited and apprehensive*

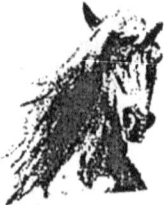

# The Sympathetic and Parasympathetic Nervous Systems

**THE NETWORK** of nerves that connect to the spinal cord and brain (the Peripheral Nervous System) has two overlapping parts. They are the somatic (under conscious control) and autonomic (self-regulating).

The **Autonomic Nervous System** normally functions outside conscious, willed control[1]; e.g. regulating breathing, digestion and pupil dilation. It has two counteracting parts, the **Sympathetic** and **Parasympathetic**.

## Sympathetic

Bodily functions speed up.

There is a high consumption of energy with some wastage of energy.

It operates when we are in **Survival Mode**[2]. This is the **Fight or Flight** response. In a frightening, life-threatening situation we have to react quickly by either attacking the threat or running away. This can be a sudden, dramatic happening or a continual sense of unease[3].

The system speeds up the heartbeat, sends more blood to the relevant muscles and enlarges the pupils of the eye to enable it to use all available light. It takes blood away from the digestive tract and sends it to the parts that need to react to the emergency. Feeding and reproduction can be part of the survival mode.

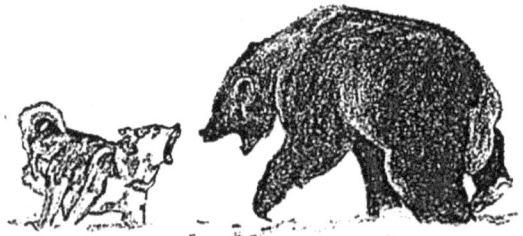

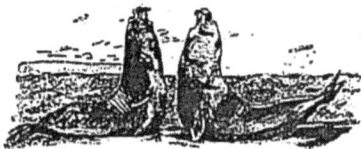

### Body Language

Movements speed up. There is an emphasis of movement in the hands, nose and face. In extreme cases there will be quick upper chest **Nose Breathing**.

The obvious example is the backward ears and flared nostrils of a horse when it is angry, frightened or threatened. One of my pupils says her husband flares his nostrils when he is angry.

This newspaper headline describes a woman defending herself in debate. *Nostrils flaring, face flushed, she snapped:*

*He's just wrong[4]*  (Please read the additional notes on Page 24)

## Parasympathetic

Bodily functions slow down.

There is a low consumption of energy with some storage of energy.

It operates when we are secure, confident and contented.

The **Four Rs** are usually used to describe its activities:
**Rest, Relax, Restore** and **Renew**.

The heart slows down and the digestive system is well supplied with blood. The pupils contract as orientation turns inwards, away from external things.

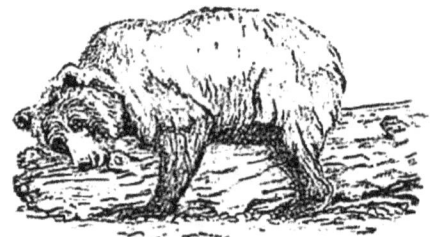

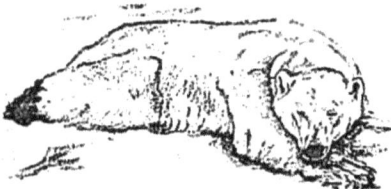

### Body Language

Movements slow down.

The hands and face become passive.

Breathing is lower down in the body. There is more diaphragm awareness and abdominal movement.

When humans and animals are deeply relaxed, **Throat Breathing (Ujjayi)** occurs naturally. It is not unusual to hear a human or dog breathing through a slightly closed throat while sleeping or dozing.

1. *It is possible to control the heart beat and other bodily functions but it takes practise and concentration. Some yogis and military personnel, for example, have trained themselves to do this (see The Psychic Warrior, by David Morehouse, ISBN 978-190-2636207).*
2. *All creatures with a backbone, e.g. humans, animals and fish, have this basic mechanism.*
3. *Swami Ambikananda, from Reading, UK, said in a workshop that she had asked a cancer specialist why so many people had cancer today. He said, Because there is too much use of the Sympathetic Nervous System.*
4. The Daily Mail, 30.1.08.

# Breath ~ Body ~ Mind ©

**Preparatory information relating to the next two sequences.** They combine movements with the breath to relieve anxiety, depression, traumatic stress and most psychological problems that affect our well-being.

**These quotations** are from videos on the **Breath, Body, Mind** website. The doctors are in discussion with students.

1. **Dr Gerbarg** is explaining why the breath is so powerful.

*Of all the autonomic functions of the body, breathing is the only one that we can voluntarily control. You can't easily, voluntarily change your heart beat or digestion, but you can change your pattern of breathing any time you wish. So breathing gives us a portal of entry where we can directly access and send messages to the interceptive system.*

*If we can figure out the language, if we can find out the code, and determine which breathing practice is going to send the messages we want to send to the higher control centres to activate them and get them to function better, then we have a chance to, very simply, change the way our emotions are regulated.*

*That's what we find over and over again when we do these studies. If you change the way people are breathing, their emotions change, their anxiety goes down, they become less depressed. We have in our hands a completely self-empowering treatment for the self-regulation of our emotions.*

*Why is breathing so powerful to the brain? Breathing is essential for our survival. If you don't get any food for a day you are still going to be alive, but if you don't breathe for 3 or 4 minutes you will die. So which messages are going to be received and paid attention to and to be given top priority? Messages from the lungs are going to override any other messages. If you can't breathe, if your airways are obstructed, your entire brain and mental apparatus has to quickly shift and figure out how to keep your airways open.*

*That's why we believe these practices can work so quickly - literally within minutes.*

2. **Dr. Brown** is explaining how breath work harmonises mind, body and spirit.

*Normally every function in your mind, body, spirit complex has a diurnal rhythm. There is an hour in the day when you do algebra and differential equations best. There's an hour or two when you are strongest physically. Every function in your mind, body, spirit has its rhythm. The thing is, these rhythms are totally chaotic and incoherent. Your energy is really incoherent.*

*When you start doing this breathing it's remarkable. You can measure how they all come together. They all align. Instead of your system being like different sections of an orchestra warming up, it becomes like an orchestra playing together and making beautiful music. Your blood-flow and your brain and your heart synchronise. So how often do your head and your heart come together? Not often, but life is much better when they do.*

For further information go to www.Breath-Body-Mind.com
They are the authors of **The Healing Power of the Breath**. 2012. Published by Shambhala.

**Please see important Additional notes on Page 24**

## The Coherent Breath

The Coherent Breath is defined as slow gentle breathing through the nose at a rate of **5 breaths per minute**. It involves **inhaling** for **6** seconds and **exhaling** for **6** seconds. Dr Brown says this breathing ratio activates the **Vagus Nerve**. This is the nerve associated with the **Parasympathetic Nervous System**. The benefits of this system can be found on the opposite page.

**There are two Coherent Breathing tracks** with piano accompaniment, on the **audio file that** comes with this book. see page 103.

# 1. The Great Harmoniser of Breath.

## Breathing Pattern
INHALE for **6** – EXHALE for **6**.
This is the **Coherent Breath,** see page **11**.

**A.** Start with the feet apart and the hands on the abdomen. **INHALE** to the count of **6** as you raise your hands above your head. The palms rotate outwards at chest level and then push upwards.

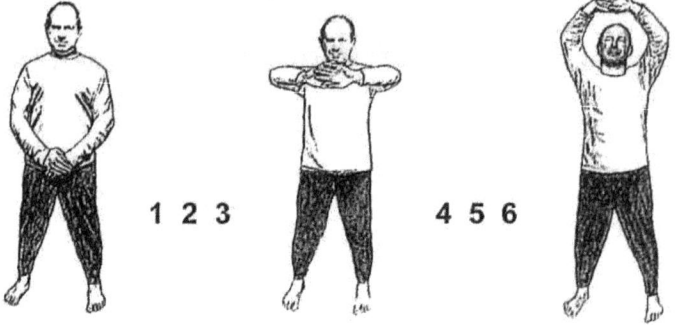

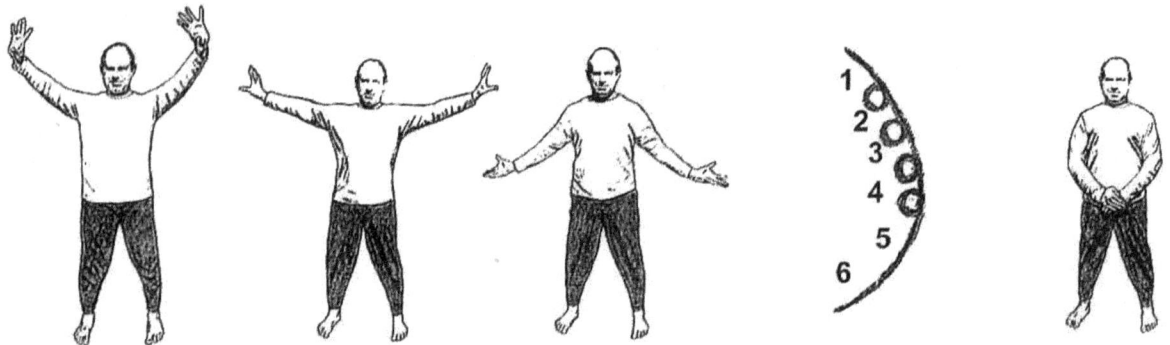

**1 2 3**      **4 5 6**

**B.** Separate the hands and prepare to lower them to the sides in a wide circle. As you **EXHALE** them down to the count of **6**, rotate your wrists **4** times and return your hands to the abdomen (see diagram above).

**C.** Repeat **A. INHALE** as you return your hands above your head.

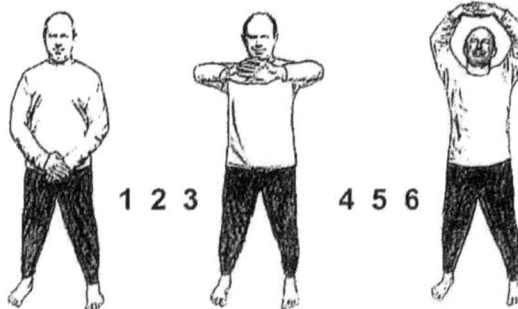

**1 2 3**      **4 5 6**

**D. EXHALE** as you circle the hands back down to the starting point with the palms facing downwards. This time, don't rotate the wrists. It is a smooth, flowing movement.

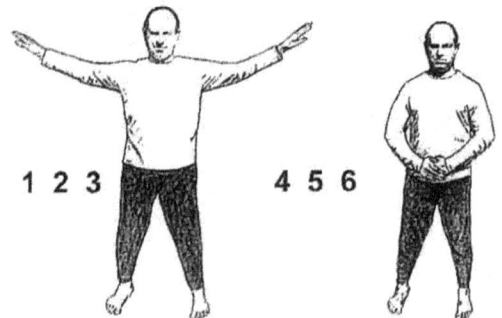

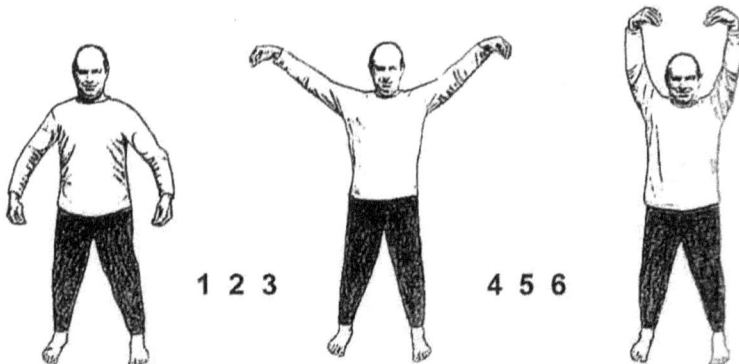

**1 2 3**      **4 5 6**

**1 2 3**      **4 5 6**

**E.** Bring your fingers and thumbs together, forming a **Crane Beak** with your hands. **INHALE** them up in a circle. The fingers turn to face each other above your head.

**F.** As you **EXHALE**, bend forwards from the hips with a flat back, bringing the hands down in front of you. Swing your hands behind you and look forwards. As you count 5 and 6, bring your feet together and bend your knees.

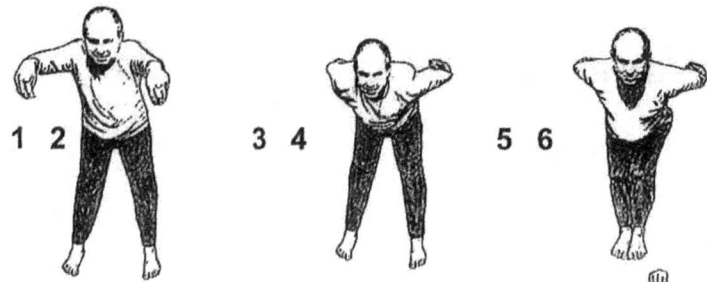

**1 2**   **3 4**   **5 6**

**G.** **INHALE** as you swing your hands forwards and sink down into a comfortable squat. Feel your weight on the heels. Gradually straighten the legs and bring the hands above your head.

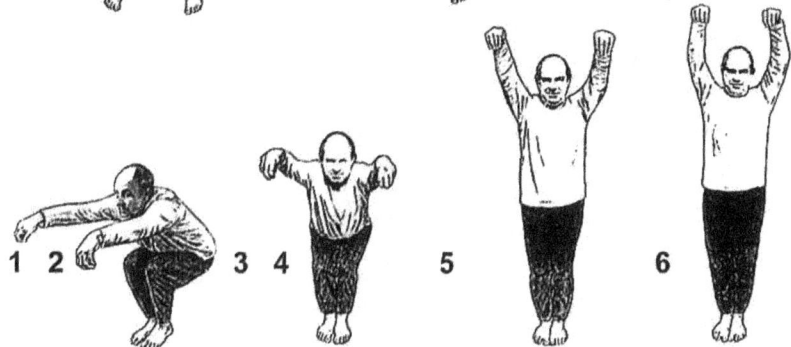

**1 2**   **3 4**   **5**   **6**

**H.** **EXHALE** as you separate your fingers and curve your hands next to your head. Stretch them forwards with the fingers overlapping[1].

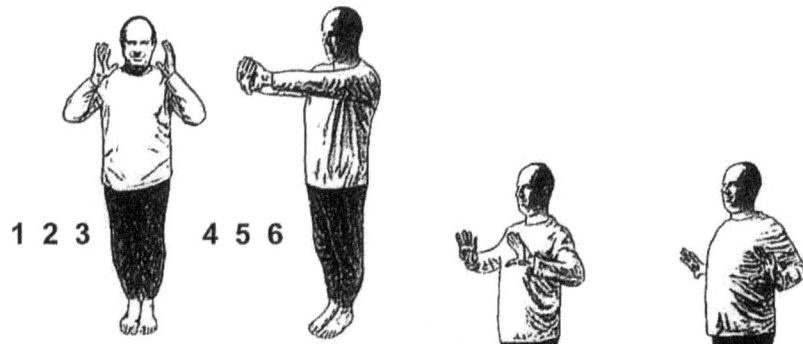

**1 2 3**   **4 5 6**

**I.** **INHALE** as you separate the hands and bring them back at shoulder height. Take the elbows as far back as you can.

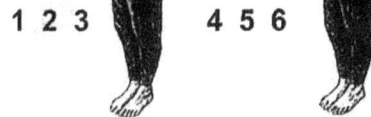

**1 2 3**   **4 5 6**

**J.** **EXHALE** as you push your palms forwards. As you count **4, 5 and 6**, step your feet apart and bring your hands back to the lower abdomen, returning to the starting point.

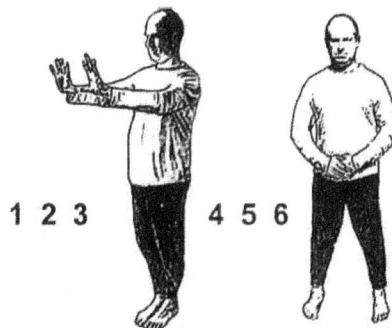

**1 2 3**   **4 5 6**

**Observations:** The same comments and cautions apply to both of these sequences. Both require regular practise. They are more difficult to memorise than you would expect and require deep concentration. This is therapeutic as it stops your mind from wandering off down leafy lanes. This level of concentration, combined with movement and the breath, creates a very powerful practice. This has been the experience of my pupils.

Daily practise of these two sequences should help to relieve anxiety, depression, traumatic stress and most psychological problems that affect our well-being.

1. The movements from H to J should feel like waves coming and going on the seashore. They can flow smoothly and gracefully like water.

## 2. QiGong Breath for Calmness, Energy and Strength.

**Breathing Pattern,** in counts roughly a second long:

**INHALE for 4 – HOLD for 4 – EXHALE for 6 – HOLD for 2**

**A.** Stand with the feet together and the knees soft and slightly bent. Place your hands on the lower abdomen with your dominant hand on top.

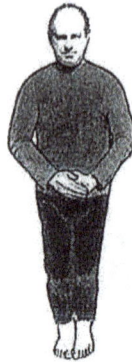

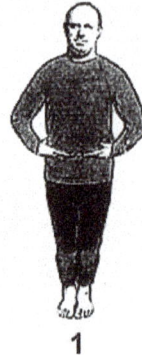

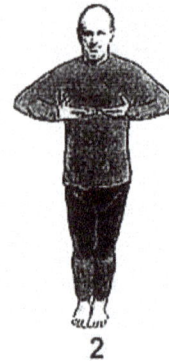

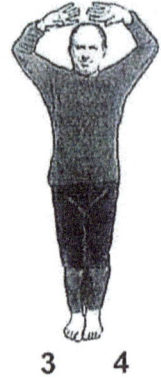

**B. INHALE** for **4** counts, starting with your palms facing upwards and bringing them above your head. It will be necessary to rotate the palms away from your body at shoulder level.

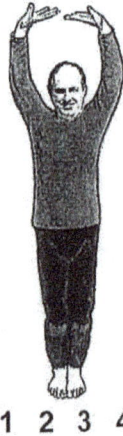

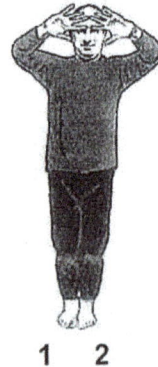

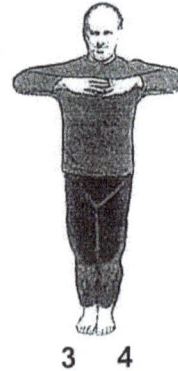

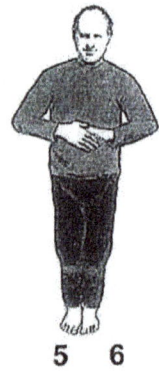

**C. HOLD** for **4** counts with the hands higher above the head, and the elbows straight.

**D. EXHALE** to the count of **6** as you bring your fingers together above your head and lower them till they are hovering just above the waist. At shoulder level your hands will rotate towards the body and your dominant hand will slide on top of the other hand.

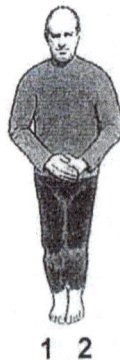

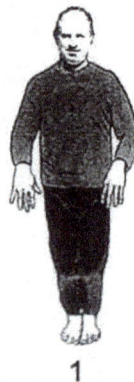

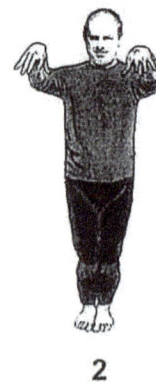

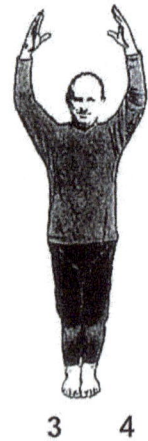

**E. HOLD¹** with your hands in the starting position (**A**) for **2** counts.

**F.** Separate your hands and, with the palms facing downwards and the arms straight, **INHALE** them above your head to the count of **4**. The hands should feel soft and heavy. The fingers will curve downwards naturally. By the fourth count your hands will be above your head with the palms facing.

**1. Caution.**
If you suffer from Chronic Obstructive Pulmonary Disease (COPD) or Emphysema, you may not want to pause for **2** counts after your exhalation in **E** and **I**. You may prefer to **EXHALE** for the count of **8**. I teach it this way in a class.

**G**. Open the arms out wide and **HOLD** for **4** counts.

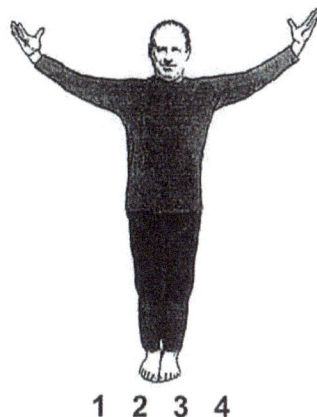

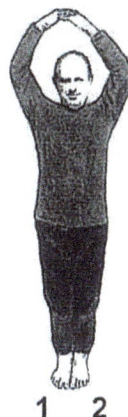

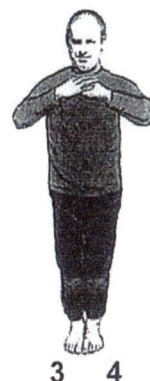

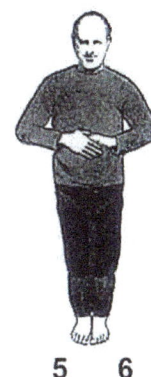

1  2  3  4          1  2          3  4          5  6

**H. EXHALE** to the count of **6** as you bring the fingers together above your head and lower the hands down, as in **D**. The dominant hand will slide on top of the other hand again.

**I**. Return to **A** and **HOLD** for **2** counts.
*Return to B and repeat*.

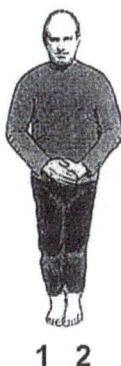

1  2

*Repeat entire sequence 16 times.*
*This takes about 5 to 7 minutes.*

## Breath ~ Body ~ Mind ©

### Practices to relieve stress, anxiety, trauma and depression

I was introduced to these powerful practices at a conference in London organised by Heather Mason of the *Minded Institute* in March, 2015. The title was *Yoga, Key to Mental Health*.
Husband and wife team, Dr Richard P. Brown MD and Dr Patricia L. Gerbarg MD, use these techniques to help victims of disasters around the world. These include the 9/11 World Trade Center attacks, the Haiti earthquake, the Horizon Gulf oil spill, slavery in the Sudan and military service trauma.
Their benefits have been demonstrated in health care practitioners, individuals with psychiatric and medical conditions, research studies and those with the disorders of Post Traumatic Stress (PTSD), Attention Deficit Hyperactivity (ADHD), mood and life stress.

> *The practices improve physical and emotional well-being and are gentle and soft and safe for most people. However, if you experience any physical discomfort, stop and relax. If the discomfort persists, seek the advice of a medical practitioner before continuing. You will need to practise these techniques every day if possible to gain maximum benefits.*

Dr Richard P. Brown MD is Associate Clinical Professor in Psychiatry at Columbia University, NY. He is an Integrative Psychiatrist, Clinical researcher, Mind-Body Qigong, Yoga and Martial Arts teacher. He developed *Breath-Body-Mind* to quickly relieve stress and trauma.
Dr Patricia L Gerbarg MD is a Harvard-trained Psychiatrist, Clinical Researcher, writer, consultant and teaches Neuroscience, integration of *Breath-Body-Mind* with Psychotherapy and natural treatments for mental health.

# Tall Person Coherent Breath Sequence

## Introduction

The original inspiration was the **Qigong *Heaven and Earth*** sequence by **Bruce Kumar Frantzis**[1]. Over the years, it has evolved to only loosely resemble the original sequence. I found it worked well with the **Coherent Breath** and my pupils found it beneficial.

> INHALE **for the count of 6**
> EXHALE **for the count pf 6**

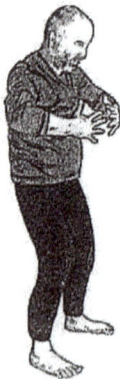

**12**. EXHALE as you straighten your arms and legs and lengthen your posture. Stretch the hands out in front as in **5**.

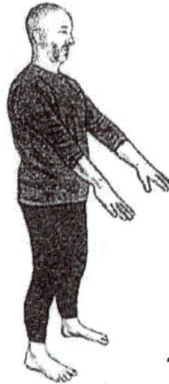

**13**. INHALE as you lower your hands to the sides and lengthen the body again into **Tall Person**.
  EXHALE and try to lengthen the body even more.
***Repeat as many times as you want to***

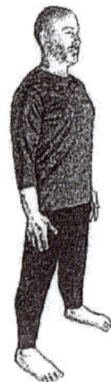

**11.** INHALE as you raise the head, lift your elbows out to the sides and turn the fingertips towards each other. Expand the chest forwards.

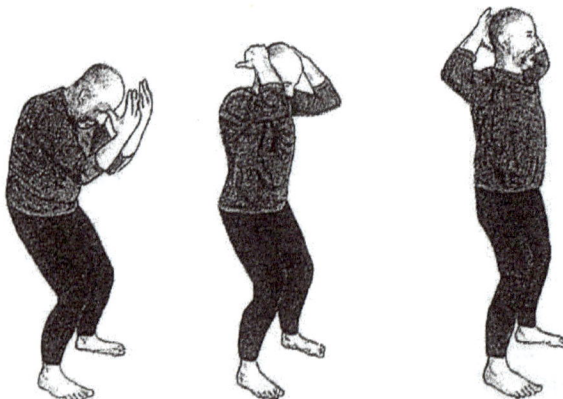

### To conclude

> **Return to normal breathing** but maintain **Tall Person** as you walk around your mat a few times. Enjoy the feeling of lightness. Try to emulate it in everyday life now and then.

**10.** EXHALE as you curve the hands over your head and bring your forearms together in front.

**9.** INHALE as you bend your knees, lean backwards a little and move your hands closer together.

**8.** EXHALE your hands behind your head, with the palms facing forwards.

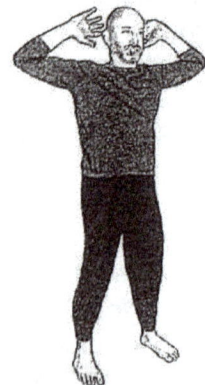

1. **Bruce Kumar Frantzis** of **Energy Arts**, USA.

**1.** Stand with your feet a hip-width apart and your hands by your sides.
INHALE as you lengthen your body to its full height in **Tall Person**. You should feel the inner arches of your feet lifting.

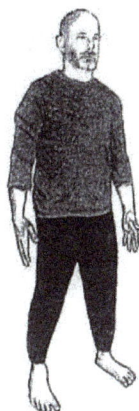

**2.** EXHALE as you bend your knees and lift your hands with the palms facing upwards and the fists clenched. Bend the elbows, keeping them close to your sides.

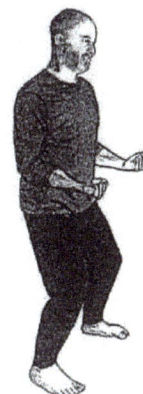

**3.** INHALE as you move the elbows back, expanding the chest.

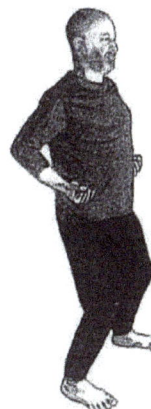

**Additional notes**
In a class, I would do the sequence at least six times, until it was memorised by most participants and could be done with the eyes closed.
  Please note that when you repeat the sequence, you will be stretching in **Tall Person** for **18** counts. In **13**, it is held for the **inhalation** and **exhalation**, and then you continue to hold it for the **inhalation** in **1**. If you find this too demanding, pause between some of the rounds.

**4.** EXHALE as you turn your palms downwards and **punch** the hands out in front.

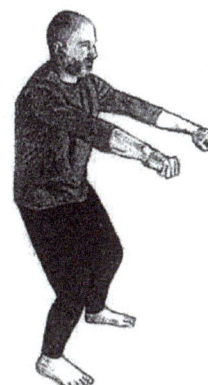

**5.** INHALE as you straighten the legs, arms and fingers out in front, as illustrated.

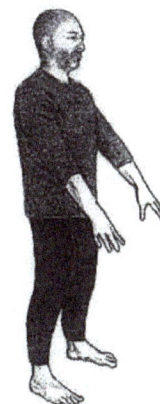

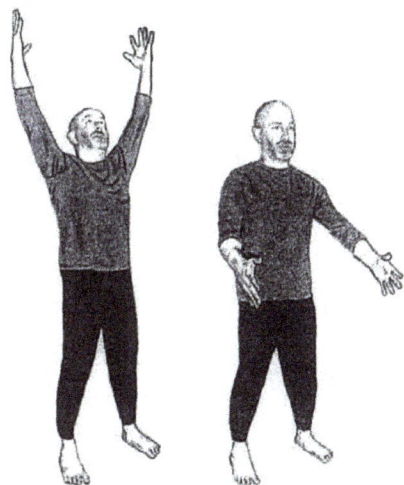

**6.** EXHALE as you stretch your body to its full height again in **Tall Person**.

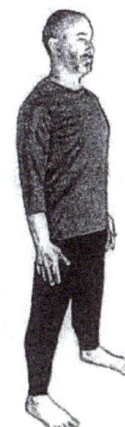

**7.** INHALE the hands up in front and stretch them above your head.

# The relevance of the Hands in our Yoga practice

The diagram below shows the **left side** of the **Sensory** and **Motor Strips** of the brain. The hands and face, especially the lips, have a large amount of space allocated to them. This explains why hand **Mudras** (the way we hold our hands during meditation and posture work) are so powerful. Each finger has a significant number of neural connections.

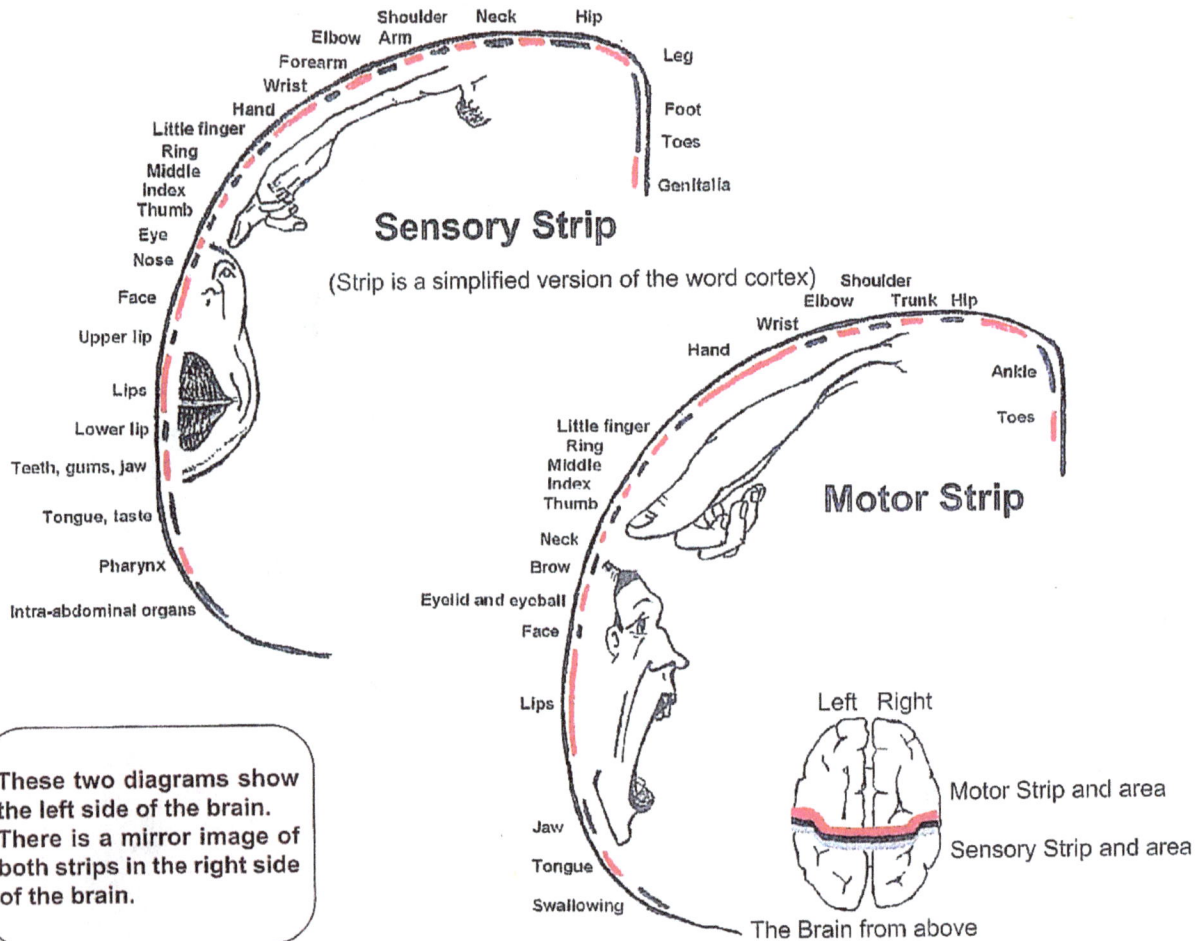

**Sensory Strip**

(Strip is a simplified version of the word cortex)

**Motor Strip**

These two diagrams show the left side of the brain. There is a mirror image of both strips in the right side of the brain.

Left   Right

Motor Strip and area

Sensory Strip and area

The Brain from above

The **left hemisphere** of the brain contols the **right hand** and the **right hemisphere** of the brain controls the **left hand**. For this reason, researchers encourage people to use both hands equally in everyday life. This will work both sides of the brain in equal ways which may benefit different aspects of life.

# The Hands in the Meridian Theory of Chinese Medicine

The oldest text of Chinese Medicine is **The Yellow Emperor's Treatise on Internal Medicine**[1]. The following information in the box comes from **The Theories of the Chakras** by Hiroshi Motoyama[2]. He says the Yellow Emperor's text is the original source of this information.

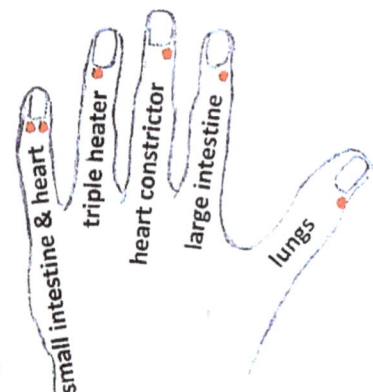

This diagram shows the **location** of the meridians in the hands. The **red spots** are the **sei points**.

*There are twelve major meridians of **ki** energy[3] which course over and through the body; most of them are related to one particular internal organ which they transverse. The terminal points of these meridians are located on the fingers and toes, and are known as **sei ('well') points**..... The meridians are virtually identical for both left and right sides.*

*The **sei points** are very important, for it is here that **ki** energy enters and leaves the meridians. The energy level at these points is said to accurately reflect the condition of the entire meridian. In cases of acute illness, acupuncture or **moxa**[4] treatment here is known to have an immediate effect........ Hand-clenching and toe-bending exercises of **pawanmuktasana**[5] directly stimulate the **sei points**, and thus promote better **ki**-energy circulation.*

In the **diagram of the hand** on the previous page, the **Triple Heater/Warmer** controls the fight, flight or freeze response, see page **10** and the **Heart Constrictor** protects the heart. It is also known as the **Guardian of the Heart**. It protects the heart from damage and disruption by excessive emotional energies generated by the other organs such as anger from the liver, fear from the kidneys and grief from the lungs.

## Modern Meridian Theory

**Meridians** are the same as **Nadis** in Yoga. They are **energy channels**.

This is a simplified version of the **Modern Meridian Theory** as presented by **Paul Grilley** in his DVD, *Yin Yoga*. His teachers researching the theory are Dr Hiroshi Motoyama, James Oschman and Stephen Birch.

***Meridians exist in water-rich phases in the connective tissue. Connective tissue is found all over the body. Life force must travel to every cell in the body. The only tissue that connects every cell of the body is connective tissue.***

Veins, arteries, nerves, etc. all have tubes and membranes. Meridians have no membranes and cannot be seen but they can be traced in little granules of **HA, Hyaluronic Acid**.

Meridians have avoided physical detection in the past because scientists did not know what to look for. Research is on-going but, so far, distinct pathways of Hyaluronic Acid have been traced in the skin, which form rivers of energy. These correspond with the established acupuncture points.

Hyaluronic Acid absorbs water. The water wraps itself around the granules. This theory suggests the Meridian System is a very different one from the Nervous System: ***Nerve impulses travel at 180 metres a second. Meridian energy travels at one metre per four seconds.***

All types of yoga postures are likely to stimulate Hyaluronic Acid. It is necessary to put appropriate stress on the joints and body components. Without some stress the body degenerates, becomes weak, and the health and energy systems are compromised. Adapting to stress makes us strong.

**1**. Dated about 2,600 BC.
**2**. The **Theories of the Chakras, Bridge to the Higher Consciousness** by **Hiroshi Motoyama**, 1925. Fourth Printing in 1995 by The Theosophical Publishing House, USA.
**3**. **Ki** energy is known as **prana**, *life force*, in yogic texts. It is called **The Force** in Star Wars movies. **Chi** and **Qui** are commonly used names in Chinese practices.
**4**. **Moxa** is a practice of burning **dried mugwort** on particular points of the body.
**5**. **Pawanmuktasana** is a group of exercises which promote the circulation of **ki** through the meridians. They release excessive wind and gases from the body.

# Finger Breathing

## Introduction

I asked Bob Camp, who has contributed many ideas for my previous books, if he had any suggestions for connecting to the breath at the beginning of a yoga class. He replied:

*I do one which can be practised in a dentist chair, when you are having your blood pressure taken or during similar scenarios.*

*Be as comfortable as you can, with perhaps fingers loosely interlocked and thumbs touching:*
*- **Breathe in** slowly - think **one** - lightly press the thumbs together.*
*- **Breathe out** slowly - think **two** - relax and release thumb pressure.*
*Continue for a few breaths.*
*- **Breathe in** slowly - think **smile**.*
*- **Breathe out** - think **relax**.*

I mentioned Bob's idea to a friend who is an acupuncturist, and she said there was a similar Qigong practice. I looked for it on the internet and came across **5 Finger Qigong for Relaxation and relief from Anxiety** by **Ananga Music**. On the same site, there was another interesting way to combine the fingers with the breath by **Pooky Knightsmith** of **Mental Health**. It was presented for children, as she aims to help children and young people, but I would expect it to be equally beneficial for older people. I haven't yet tried it out on my pupils because, as I write, we are in the 2020 coronavirus lockdown. Personally, I found it intriguing and comforting. I also found it worked well with the **Coherent Breath**.

## 1. Sei (or Well) Point Breathing

When I read Bob Camp's suggestion above, I immediately thought of the diagram at the bottom of page **18**. You will need to read the information about it before starting this method. I tried my idea out in classes and it seemed to be appreciated.

## The Method

Bring the **Sei** points of the **thumbs** together, on the outsides and just underneath the nails, as illustrated. Breathe slowly and deeply.

**INHALE** count **one** and push the **Sei** points together gently.
**EXHALE** and think **Aum (Om)** and release the pressure.
**Repeat** all the way up to **five**
**Reverse** the counting, repeating **five** and working through to **one**.

After the ten breaths, move on to the **Sei** points of your **index** finger and repeat the procedure.

Continue moving on to the other fingers. When you get to the **ring** fingers, you will have to adjust your hand positions because the **Sei** points are on the other side of the fingers.

There are two **Sei** points on the **little** fingers, so have one palm facing up and the other down and bring the four points together, as illustrated.

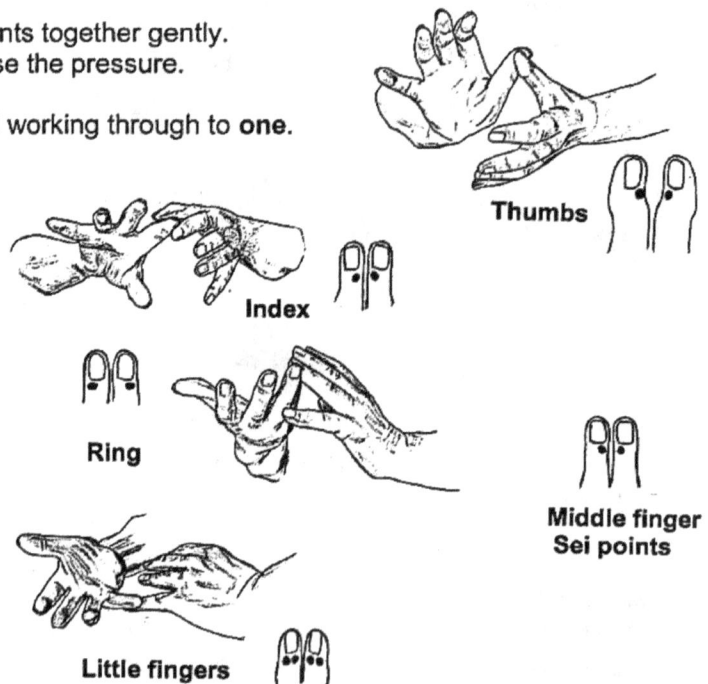

Thumbs

Index

Ring

Middle finger Sei points

Little fingers

## Additional notes

If you want a shorter practice, miss out the reverse counting and just do the five breaths per pair of fingers.
**Caution** Do not apply too much pressure. There are complex energies in these locations. Stop the practise if it appears to be having a negative effect on you.

**Practitioners are usually advised** to be in a **comfortable seated position** when working with the breath. As so many people have jobs which involve sitting down most of the time, an **alternative posture is necessary** for the body. It is possible to feel quite relaxed when you are standing, if your posture is well aligned. A compromise would be to stand with your back against a wall. If you feel this relates to you personally, try these **Finger Breathing** methods standing up.

## 2. Five Finger Breathing

This is inspired by **5 Finger Qigong** mentioned in the introduction, but I am adding the counting element, a variation, and making minor changes. In the video it says hold each combination of fingers for **one minute**. I'm suggesting breathing **5** times a minute and counting the breaths instead of counting minutes. This involves:

**Inhaling** for 6 and **exhaling** for 6 ---- or **inhaling** for 4 and **exhaling** for 8   x 5 = 60 seconds

**To make the counting easier**, try changing the count each time you **inhale**, e.g.:

| 1st INHALE | EXHALE | 2nd INHALE | EXHALE | 3rd INHALE etc. |
|---|---|---|---|---|
| 1 2 3 4 5 6 | 1 2 3 4 5 6 | 2 2 3 4 5 6 | 1 2 3 4 5 6 | 3 2 3 4 5 6 |

## The Method
Make a circular shape with the **thumbs** and **index fingers** of both hands. Rest the hands on your thighs with the palms facing upwards. **Press the tips** of your **thumbs** and **index fingers together** creating a subtle, gentle pressure. Maintain the pressure for **5** breaths, using one of the breathing ratios above.

After the five breaths, move to the **thumbs** and **middle fingers** for another five breaths, applying the pressure, as before.

Repeat the procedure with the **ring** and **little** fingers.

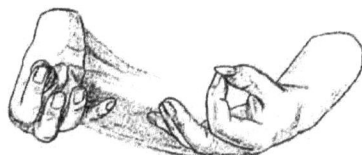 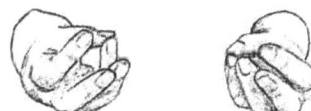

## Variation
With the wrists lightly resting on the abdomen, bring the tips of the fingers of both hands together. The **index** fingers and **thumbs** make a **Heart shape**. This is **Hakini** mudra.

You can do this practice sitting, standing or lying on your back.

**Start** by pressing the **thumbs** together for **5** breaths, counting as above. Then move onto the **index** fingers and press them together for one minute. You can maintain a very gentle pressure on the **thumbs** throughout if you choose.

Move on in the same way, through the other three fingers.

### Additional notes
You can use this mudra to enhance your meditation. **Inhale** as you apply pressure to pairs of fingers and release it as you **exhale**.

I have noticed politicians using this mudra when in conversations. To learn more about this very interesting mudra go to:

easyayurveda.com/2019/12/12/hakini-mudra/

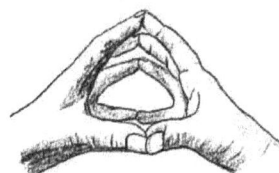

**Hakini Mudra**

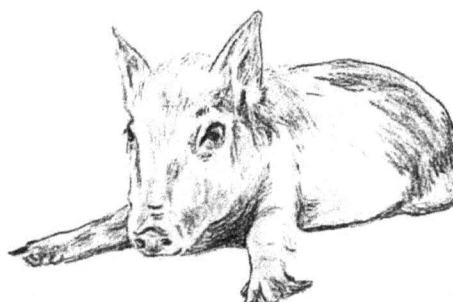

## Up and Down Finger Breathing

**Pooky Knightsmith** doesn't use my counting method in her video or my name for it. You can try it out both ways, with or without counting. **If you do count**, you can use the same ratios as before but **do not pause** after each **inhalation** and **exhalation**.
This is the way **Pooky does it**:

## The Method

Hold one hand out in front with the palm facing forwards. Spread the fingers out. Place one finger of the other hand (she uses the index finger) at the base of the thumb, on the outside.

INHALE slowly as you slide the finger along the side of the thumb to the top. **Pause** briefly.
EXHALE slowly as you slide the finger down the other side of the thumb, to the area between the thumb and index finger. **Pause** briefly.
INHALE as you slide the finger up the index finger. **Pause**. EXHALE down the other side. **Pause**.
*Repeat the procedure, breathing up and down the other three fingers*.

When you have **exhaled** down the outside of the little finger, continue sliding along the bottom of your hand, back to the place you started from, at the bottom of the outside of your thumb.
*Repeat as many times as you want to*.
**Pooky** doesn't say anything about changing hands, but I'm sure you can if you want to.

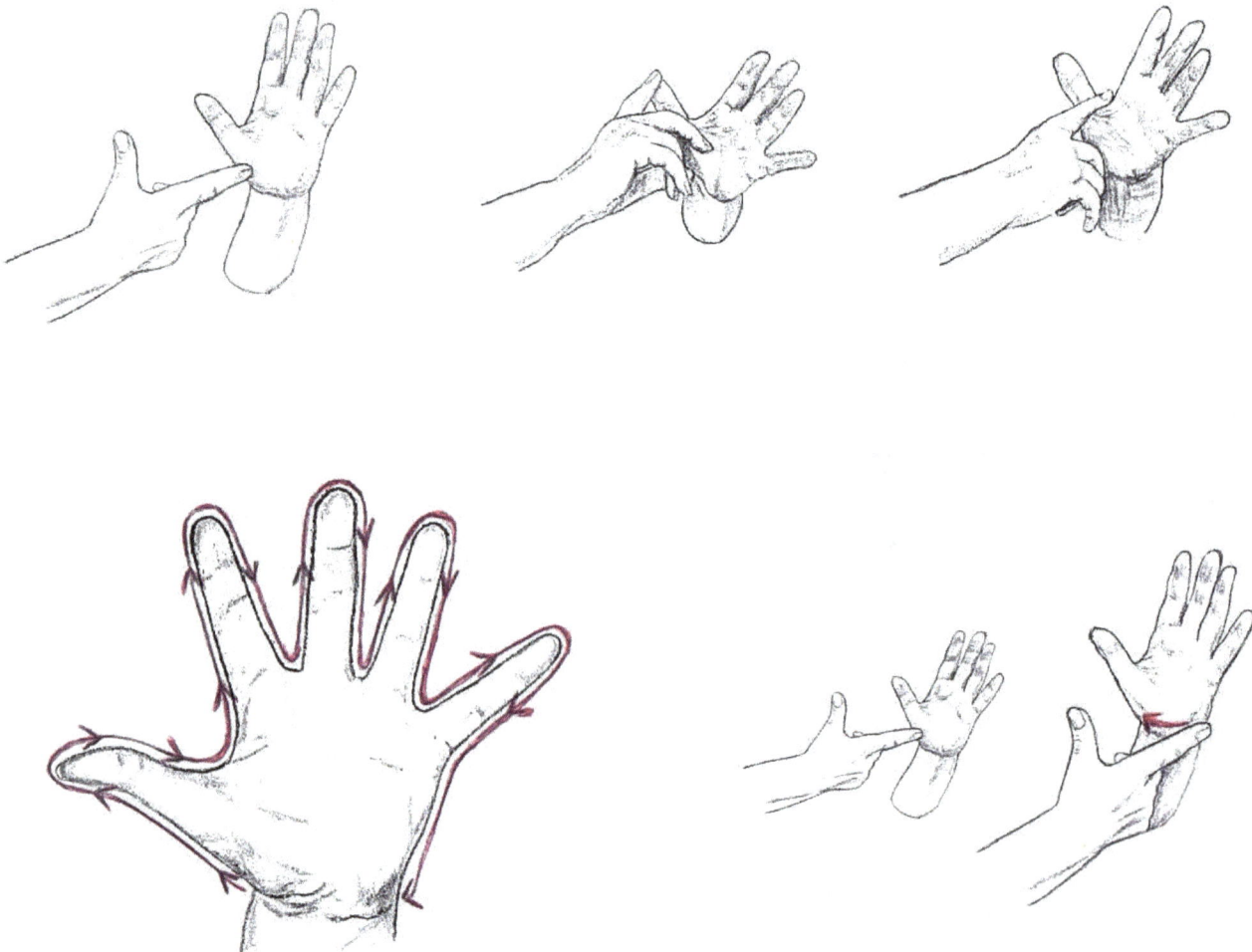

# Nose and Throat Breathing

This section is inspired by **Sophie Gabriel's** book, ***Breath for Life***[1]. She is not a yoga teacher but she is familiar with yogic breathing and praises its effectiveness. She teaches correct breathing techniques from the perspective of personal well-being.

She uses the concept of Nose and Throat Breathing. This input led me to make the connection between **Nose Breathing** and the **Sympathetic Nervous System** and **Throat Breathing** and the **Parasympathetic Nervous System**, see page **10**

In **Nose Breathing** the sensations are felt in the nose.
In **Throat Breathing** they are felt in the throat.

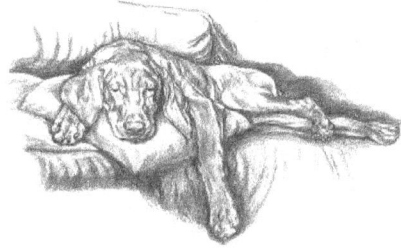

## Throat Breathing

This is called **Ujjayi** in **Yoga** and **Ibuki** in **Karate**.

Here are some quotations from Sophie Gabriel's book:

*Throat breathing is the kind of breathing that happens naturally when good quality deep breathing occurs ... The sound also gives you the opportunity to monitor and observe the quality and duration of your breathing.*

*When I am teaching someone to breathe a good quality breath, the first concept I teach is how to throat breath, and I do not continue with the rest of the training until they have grasped it.*

Other names for **Ujjayi** are Victorious Breath[2], Ocean Sounding Breath, Psychic Breath (because of the effect it has on the mind) and I have even heard it called Darth Vader Breath. I am adding Steam Engine Breath and Dozy Dog Breath, after observing that my brothers dog Rolo, a chocolate Labrador, is an excellent ujjayi breather when he is very relaxed.

Although most people do ujjayi naturally when they are sleeping, or concentrating and relaxing deeply, I find that some of my pupils are timid, awkward ujjayi breathers and don't adjust well to producing the sound in class. In contrast, some pupils find it so easy and beneficial that they tend to do it to some degree (loudly or softly) for most of the class. I personally find it so beneficial that I make a point of doing it most of the day (you can do it silently but still put the emphasis on the throat) as a way of inducing the parasympathetic nervous system and saving energy.

Here are some quotations from the ***Hatha Yoga Pradipika***[3].

*The practice of ujjayi is so simple that it can be done in any position and anywhere ... It helps relax the physical body and the mind, and develops awareness of the subtle body and psychic sensitivity. Ujjayi promotes internalization of the senses and pratyahara*[4].

*Ujjayi is especially recommended for people who have insomnia and mental tension. It is a must in the yogic management of heart disease. However, anyone with high bold pressure must first correct their condition before taking up the practice.*

### Method

The original method was making the noise in the throat while inhaling through both nostrils, retaining the breath and then exhaling quietly and slowly through the left nostril. These are slightly simplified quotes from the *Hatha Yoga Pradipika*.

*Closing the mouth, draw in the breath through both nostrils till the breath fills the space from the throat to the heart with the noise. Perform kumbhaka (pause and hold the breath) and exhale through the left nostril ... This is called ujjayi and it can be done while moving, standing, sitting or walking.*

During the last century, some teachers discovered the benefits of using ujjayi during sequential posture work. They omitted the pause and made the noise on inhalation and exhalation and exhaled through both nostrils. This is now the accepted practice in yoga classes.

The noise is made by gently constricting the opening of the throat and creating some resistance to the passage of air. It cannot be made without engaging with the diaphragm. The diaphragm expands downwards to draw the air in through a slightly closed throat. Some teachers think it causes tension in the throat and avoid it, but if it is done gently, using our natural technique, it should have the opposite effect.

1. Breath for Life. Basic Health Publications, Inc. ISBN 1-59120-002-4
2. *Ujji* is the root which means 'to conquer' or 'acquire by contest'.
3. From the Hatha Yoga Pradipika. *Commentary by Swami Muktibodhananda Saraswati, under the guidance of Swami Satyananda Sararwati.* Bihar School of Yoga.
4. The fifth stage in Patanjali's Eight Limbs of Raja Yoga. It is the process of *disconnecting from the outside world* and *taking the senses inwards* before concentration and meditation.

# Additional notes about the Coherent Breath

After I read **Stephen Elliott's** book **The New Science of Breath**[1], I felt clarification was necessary. I had wrongly assumed that the **Coherent Breath**, **inhaling** for the count of **6** and exhaling for the count of **6** (breathing **five times a minute**) was to access the **Parasympathetic** nervous system. Steve Elliott says this rate of breathing accesses the **mid-point** between the **Sympathetic** (which speeds up) and **Parasympathetic** (which slows down) nervous systems. It is like being in neutral gear when driving a car.

Although **inhaling** for the count of **4** and **exhaling** for the count of **8** is also breathing **five times a minute**, it is not the **mid-point** between the nervous systems. It verges more towards the **Parasympathetic** nervous system. The heart slows down as you exhale.

At a workshop in 2019 organised by the Minded Institute, Dr. Richard Brown said that breathing five times a minute is for people of average height. Shorter people, this includes children, need to increase the rate and very tall people need to reduce it to achieve the same neutral point in the **Autonomic Nervous System**. The rate for children is **ten** times a minute, **inhaling** for **3** seconds and **exhaling** for **3** seconds. They will be able to use the soundtrack as they will be inhaling and exhaling in six seconds. For tall people, the ratio is **4.5** breaths per minute which is only a little slower than five times a minute. They should still find the **6/6** ratio beneficial.

The information on page **10** describes the extremes of the **Autonomic** nervous systems.
You could speculate that the **Sympathetic** system was the *bad guy* that stresses us out, but most of us need it to get out of bed in the morning and to access motivation and courage. It mobilises energy.

1. **Stephen Elliott** is credited with the development and articulation of the **Coherent Breathing** method. **The New Science of Breath**, 2005, by **Stephen Elliott** and **Dee Edmonson, RN**, is published by **Coherence Publishing**.

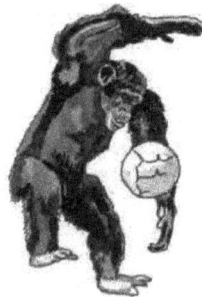

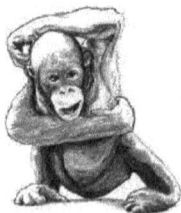

# Introduction to T L C Breathing
## Tender Loving Care Breathing

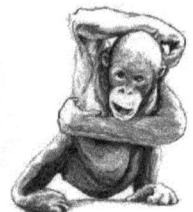

### Sources of ideas in this sequence
This is another sequence that has its roots in one of Tasha's Glastonbury yoga retreats[1]. We did **1 - 3** and massages similar to **4 - 7** and then **Hugs**, as in **14**. Later I thought of combining these and other movements with the **Coherent Breath** (see page **11** and above).
Concentrating on the breath while massaging is not a new idea. **Swami Sivananda** says in his book, **Health and Long Life**[2]; *When you do massage, repeat the name of the Lord and practise Pranayama and Kumbhak*[3].

**7** and the **Neck Stretch** in **8** are inspired by ideas in **Chair Yoga** by **Kristin Mcgee**[4]. The **Neck Massage** in **8** and others up to **13**, I put together myself. The **Peace Salutation**, **15**, is from videos by **Erin Sampson** of **Five Parks Yoga**. I sometimes end my classes with it.

## Historical notes on Self Massage

Massage is described in the oldest Hindu and Chinese books. People used their hands to rub away their aches and pains before there were modern-day medication and medical practitioners.

There was a traditional Asian self-massage called **Do-in**. This is described and illustrated by **Kristine Kaoverii Weber** in her book **Healing Self Massage**[5]. She says: *Taoist monks were the first to systemize the self-healing instinct and called their method Tao-Yin ('The way' or 'Gentle approach')..... The term became 'do-in' in Japanese, and today this technique is used as a form of self-help shiatsu*[6].

I came across this book after I had developed my sequence so it is not influenced by it, but some of the ideas are inevitably similar.

Tibetan Healing also has a long tradition of self-massage. There is an Egyptian wall painting/mural (c. 2345 to 2181 BC) in Ankhmahar. The scene depicts a hand massage being given. It is possible that they developed self-massage as well. I am not aware of any more historical evidence but it is probable that many cultures around the world developed their own types of massage.

## Additional notes

I have kept the instructions and explanations at a very basic level in this sequence. I could have written more about the benefits and physiology, but too much information and too many words can detract from the simple enjoyment of touching, stroking and massaging.

I searched the internet for relevant ideas and found some advice in a YouTube video by **Spencer** titled **Common Massage Mistakes Beginner Therapists Make**. His first two points were: *Don't go too deep too quickly* and *Don't use the thumbs too much*.

**Swami Sivananda** says, in the book mentioned on page **24**: *Massage should not be merely applying friction. It may be very vigorous in strong persons. It must be gentle in persons of delicate health.* So be sensitive about the amount of pressure you use in the movements. If you feel your constitution can accommodate strong **tapping** in **4 - 6**, experiment but proceed with caution. Discover how much pressure it is safe to use.

Sometimes light, gentle strokes and massaging can be as relaxing and beneficial as stronger ones. If you are unwell, have a weak constitution or simply feel like a gentle massage, you can experiment using less pressure and light, stroking movements throughout this sequence.

**Tapping**: Some people may need to have this term clarified. It involves applying pressure/friction, mostly to the muscles, with a clenched fist. This is done by holding the fist or fists, a short distance away from the selected area and then tapping it with the chosen amount of pressure. The fists do not linger on the area. They bounce off ready for the next tap. It will be repeated in the same place a few times until the benefits have been felt. It stimulates the skin and muscles and promotes the flow of blood and lymph.

I have started to use **TLC Breathing** at the beginning of a **Restorative Class**. You can sit on the bolsters usually used in this class. This sequence can take between 15 minutes and half an hour to do. I find Restorative classes are very popular and I like to do 3 or 4 weeks of them each year.

**Caution**: In the **Neck Stretch (8)**, do not apply too much pressure on your neck. Let the weight of your arms and hands produce the stretch without forcing it. If you have neck problems, proceed with caution and stop if there is any discomfort.

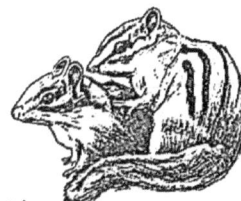

1. See information about **Tasha** in the **Introduction to the Earth Flow** on page 41.
2. **Health and Long Life** by **Swami Sivananda**, 1945, published by the Divine Life Society, Rishikesh.
3. **The Lord** probably means any Deity or representation of the **Divine Energy** that you personally identify with. It could be female, e.g., Durga or Saraswati. **Pranayama** is developing the full potential of the breath (see Glossary). **Kumbhak** means breath retention, usually after the inhalation. *Kumbha* means *pot* in Sanskrit. It compares the torso to a vessel full of air.
4. Published in US, 2017 by Harper Collins and in UK, 2017, by Piatkus. ISBN 978-0-349-41608-3
5. This is published by **Collins and Brown**, 2005, ISBN: 1-84340-211-4
6. **Shiatsu** is a modern Japanese therapy, with ancient roots in Chinese medicine; it fuses traditional Eastern practices with Western techniques of osteopathy.

# T L C Breathing
## Tender Loving Care Breathing

### 1. Massaging the Legs

Stand with the feet slightly apart. Rest your fingers on the outside of your ankles and the thumbs on the front of the legs.

INHALE to the count of **6** as you slide the fingers up the back of the calves. Apply comfortable pressure on the calves and the front of the legs.

EXHALE to the count of **6** as you move the heels of the hands around to just below your knees and slide them down the lower legs. The thumbs are on the inside of the legs and the fingers on the outside.

*Repeat about five times*.

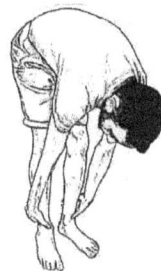

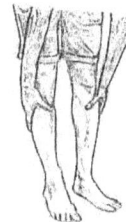

2. Use the same hand movements, but this time slide all the way up the legs to the top of the thighs and down again. INHALE up and EXHALE down, both to the count of **6**.

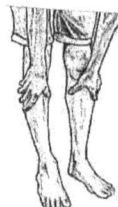

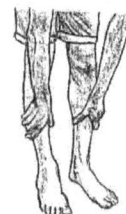

### 3. Massaging the Heels and Soles of the Feet

Sit on a minimum of two yoga blocks with your legs along the sides, as illustrated. If your knees complain, use four blocks or a bolster with cushions.

INHALE-6 as you take your left hand across to your right then sweep it up over the head and down to the left foot.

EXHALE-6 as you massage your left heel and sole of the foot. **Continue with this breathing ratio** as you massage the heel with the fingers and thumbs and use the knuckles to slide up and down the soles of the feet.

*Continue for about five breaths*, massaging as deeply as you can.

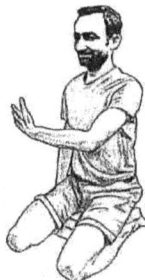

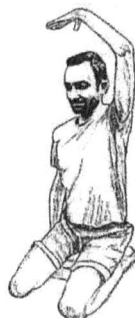

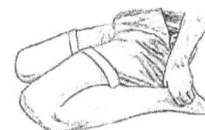

### 4. Massaging and Tapping the Back

Place the knuckles on either side of your back, just below the waist. You are going to massage the back, slowly making circles with your knuckles. INHALE-6 for half the circle and EXHALE-6 for the other half.

Spend some time exploring your back from the buttocks and lower spine to the upper rib cage, muscles at the side of the spine and the kidneys. The hands keep to their own sides of the back.

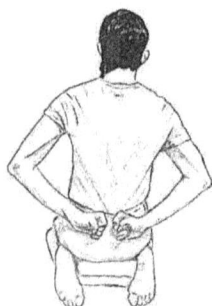

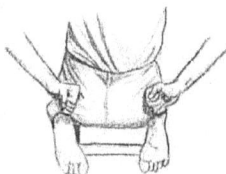

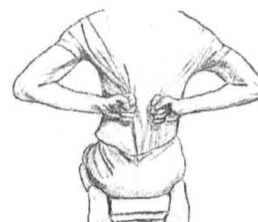

**When you are ready**, change to tapping your back. Choose an appropriate amount of pressure for your constitution. Never cause discomfort.

INHALE-6,, as you tap your back six times with both hands. Repeat this when you EXHALE.
Move around your back as in **4**.

**5.** Repeat **3** on the right side. INHALE-6 the right hand up and over the head to the left and down to the right foot. Continue to massage the heel and sole of the foot as in **3** using the **6-6** breathing ratio.

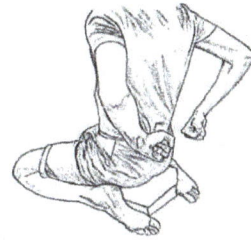

### 6. Massaging and Tapping the Abdomen

Lean backwards a little, increasing the distance between the **pubic bone** and the **sternum**. Change your sitting position if you need to. You can sit in **Easy Pose** with the legs crossed or move to a chair.

Now massage the **abdomen**, **liver** and **stomach** in the same way that you massaged the back in **4**. When you massage above the waist, you can make oblong shapes instead of circles. Keep counting in **6**s.

Now tap or thump the **abdomen** in the same way as you tapped your back. You can include the hollows at the tops of the thighs; the **groins**. Continue with the same counting.

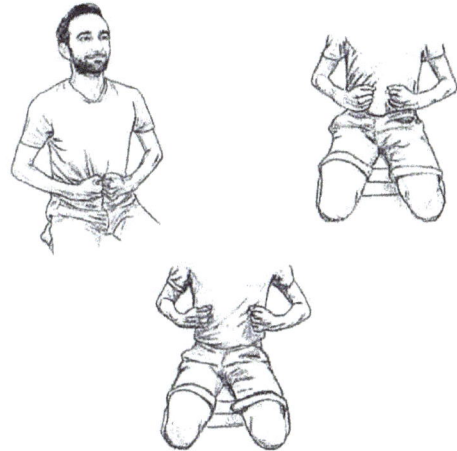

### 7. Massaging the Front of the Neck and Jaw

You can move to a chair now if you haven't done so already.
Make fists with your hands. You are going to massage the front of your neck and jaw with your knuckles. Start with them about six inches apart, resting on the **collar bones** bellow the ears. INHALE-6 before you move.
EXHALE-6 as you slide the knuckles up the sides of your neck and jaw applying an appropriate amount of pressure. INHALE-6 . For the first **4** counts flick your hands out in front with the palms upwards, fingers spread out wide and the little fingers touching. For the last **2** counts return the hands to the **collarbones**. You can work your way inwards so you eventually come up with the hands touching in the middle and slide up over the chin.

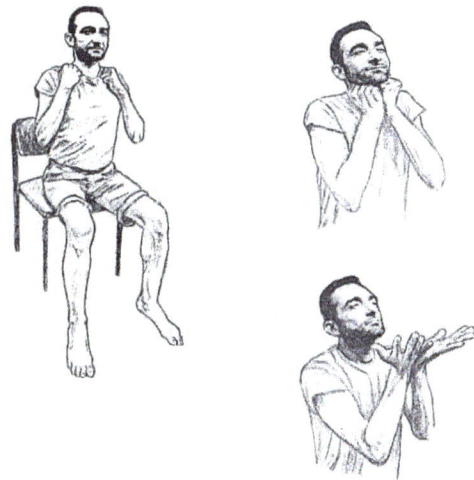

### 8. Neck Stretch and Massage

See the **Caution** on page **74** before proceeding.
Change the breathing to a **4/8** ratio here so you can develop a feel for it.
Interlock your hands on the back of your head. INHALE-4 as you open out the elbows and lean back a little. EXHALE-8 as you lower your head, stretching the back of your neck and bringing the elbows towards each other in front. *Repeat as many times as you want to.*

Rest your fingers on the back of your head just behind the ears. INHALE-4 as you open out the elbows as above and lean back a little. EXHALE-8 as you lower the head and massage the back of your neck with both hands. *Repeat as above.*

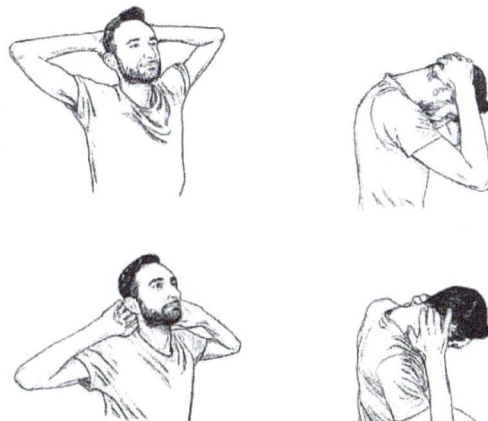

28

## 9. Massaging the Temples and Forehead

**Temple Circling.** Concentrate on the area between the end of the eyebrows and the ears, see diagram on page **31**. Move your knuckles or fingertips (this will be the three middle fingers) slowly in small circles, keeping to the **4/8** breathing ratio. *Repeat at least five times and then change direction.*

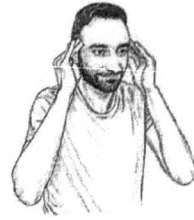

**Forehead Circling.** With the palms of your hands lightly touching your face and the little fingers touching, start to make small circles moving out towards the **Temples** on each side. Breathe as above. One hand moves **clockwise** and the other **anticlockwise**. When you reach the side of the **forehead**, change direction and slowly circle back to the central starting position. You will make about six circles in each direction. As this is so relaxing *you may want to repeat it.*

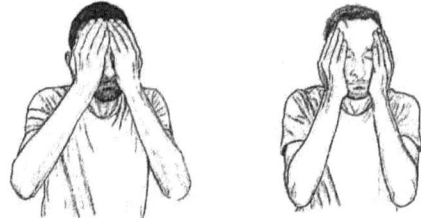

## 10. Massaging your Eyebrows and Jaw

Rest your fingertips on either side of your chin, as illustrated. **INHALE-4** as you slide your fingers up either side of your mouth and over the bony part of your nose to the area between the **eyebrows**. Touch the nostrils gently so that you do not interfere with the breathing. **EXHALE-8** as you move the fingers along the **eyebrows**. Stroke along the outside of the face, close to the ears and down to the **jaw**. Slide the fingers along the **jaw** back to the starting point, including a few circular massaging movements.
*Repeat as many times as you want to.*

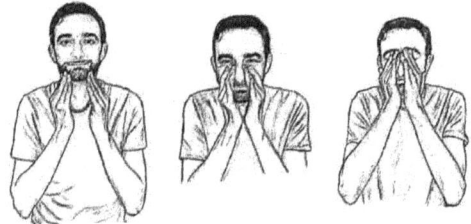

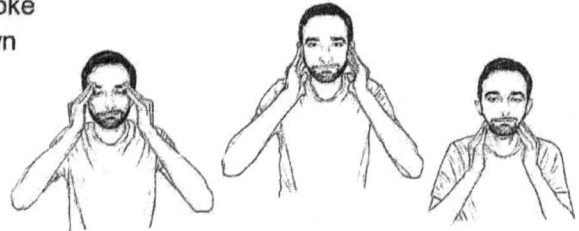

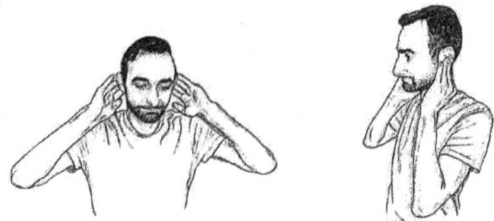

## 11. Massaging your Ears

Place your three middle finger tips behind your earlobes. **INHALE-4** as you slide your fingers around the backs of your **ears** to the top. **EXHALE-8** as you slide your fingers round the outside of your **ears** to the **earlobe**. You can also explore the front of your ear and massage the earlobe on subsequent **exhalations**.
*Repeat as many times as you want to.*

## 12. Massaging the Scalp

This may require some experimentation. You may want to change the direction of your circles when you move to different parts of the head. You can use the fingertips and apply the amount of pressure that seems right for you personally. Sometimes you can use the thumbs as well. As you **INHALE-4**, push the scalp up and towards the centre of the head. As you **EXHALE-8**, complete the circle moving down and round.

Take your time to explore the scalp, down to the base of the skull, behind the ears and the front and top of the head. *Continue for as long as you want to.*

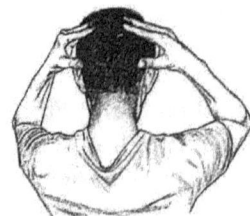

### 13. Arm, Hand and Shoulder Massage

Place the palm of your right hand on your right knee and your left hand on the right shoulder.  INHALE-4 as you slide your left hand down the right arm to the fingertips, applying as much pressure as you choose.  EXHALE-8 as you rotate the palm upwards and slide the left hand up the inside of your hand and arm to the shoulder.

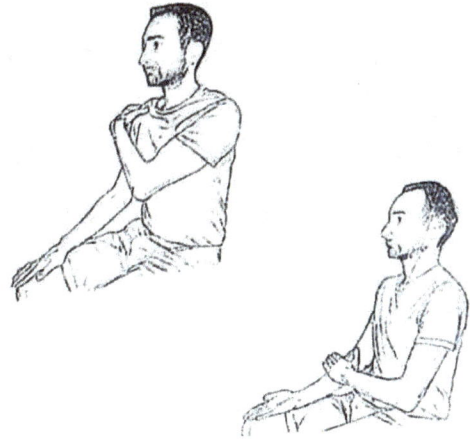

**After a few breaths** you can change over:
With the palm facing upwards, INHALE-4  up the arm, from fingers to shoulder. EXHALE-8  as you rotate the palm downwards and slide all the way down the arm to the fingers. *Repeat a few times.*
*Change arms and repeat.*

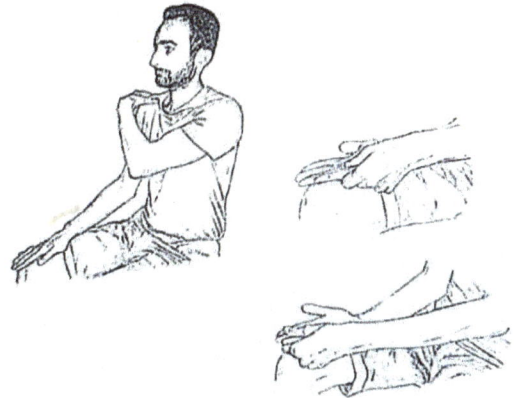

### Massaging the Hands and Shoulders

Return to the right palm resting on the right knee.  Place the left hand on top of the right hand. INHALE-4  as you slide the left hand up to the shoulder.  EXHALE-8 as you massage the right shoulder with the left hand.
INHALE-4 as you rotate the right palm upwards and slide the left hand down towards it.
EXHALE-8 as you massage the right hand.
When you massage the hand, sometimes you can concentrate on the fingers and sometimes the palm or thumb.
*Rotate the palm downwards and repeat a few times.*
*Change arms and repeat.*

### 14. Hugs

Sit up straight and  INHALE-4 as you lift and open your arms. Lift the **Heart Centre** and smile down into it.
EXHALE-8 as you lower your head a little, round your back and wrap your arms around yourself.  One hand will go on the opposite rib cage and the other on the opposite shoulder.
**Give yourself a good hug.**
*Change the arms over* each time you EXHALE
*Continue for as long as you want to.*

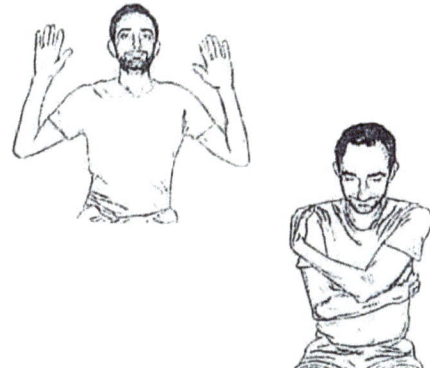

### 15.  Conclude with the Peace Salutation

*May peace be in your **thoughts**, may peace be in your **words**, may peace be in your **heart**.*

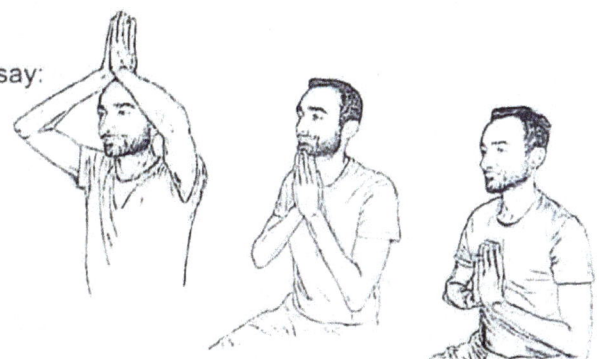

Place your hands in **Prayer** on top of your head and say:
*May peace be in your **thoughts**.*

Move your hands down to the **Throat Centre**:
*May peace be in your **words**.*

Move your hands down to the **Heart Centre**:
*May peace be in your **heart**.*

# Introduction to Warm Ups

This is divided into two sections: Thoppukaranam or Super Brain Yoga and Sukshma Vyayama or Warm-ups.
Both are appropriate for morning workouts or the beginning of a yoga class. They would also be advantageous for anybody seeking to improve their health and mental well-being.

Although I have been teaching and learning about yoga for more than 20 years, I had never come across these practices, but when I put *Thoppukaranam/Super Brain Yoga*, *Sukshma Vyayama* and *Sthula Vyayama*[1] into my search engine, I discovered rivers of information and videos.

## The Sources

I was introduced to these **Warm Ups** by Robert Moses[2] at a Hatha Intensive course in the Himalayas in 2018. I return to them on a regular basis for three consecutive weeks and my pupils find them intriguing and beneficial. Robert begins all his classes with them.

**Thoppukaranam** is a Tamil (southern Indian) term which means *to hold the ears*. The practice has been evident in Indian culture from ancient times. It was traditionally practised in the early morning facing the east (the sun). It was used to salute Lord Ganesha[3], whilst simultaneously tuning the nervous system and warming the body.
It was taught to all children in the ancient Gurukula Systems to stimulate and energize the brain and its functions. It spread to many countries. Unfortunately, it became associated with punishment, possibly because it proved efficient at improving bad behaviour and under the influence of western colonialism.

> In eastern medicine, the outer portion of the ear is viewed as a micro-system representing the entire body. According to neurologist Dr. Paul Nogier, MD, the ear corresponds to the inverted foetus curled in the womb. Points of the ear correspond with specific areas of the body and the ear lobe corresponds to the head. Consequently, massage of these points can produce therapeutic benefits to the brain.

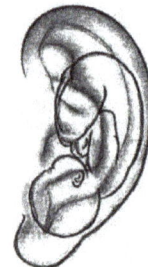

## Interpretation, Observations and Research

In modern times, this practice has been re-popularized by some enthusiasts and promoted in many parts of the world as **Super Brain Yoga**.
Dr. Eric Robins, a medical doctor from Los Angeles, calls it *a fast, simple, drug-free method of increasing mental energy* and prescribes it to his patients. He speaks of one student who raised his grades from C's to A's in a space of one semester.
Occupational therapist Raina Koterba says the effect on one autistic seven-year-old boy was immediate and dramatic. Before learning the exercise, the boy had frequent episodes of violence, including kicking, biting, punching and head-butting, *but since he started the exercise he has not had one outburst*.
Denise Peak, a high school teacher of students with learning disabilities including autism and Aspergers Syndrome, has had very encouraging results. She says, *I think this might be the key to help unlock these children*.
Yale neurobiology researcher Dr. Eugenius Yang, Jr. says the practice stimulates neural pathways in the brain by activating acupuncture points on the earlobes and synchronizes the right and left hemispheres of the brain, as demonstrated by EEG (electroencephalograph) scans. *I do it every day*, he said. He has prescribed this for patients with Alzheimer's and children with autism and Attention Deficit Hyperactivity Disorder. **All these comments** come from a video, *What is Super Brain Yoga* by **Dr Eric Robin**.

1. **Sukshma** means *fine and delicate*, **Sthula** means *dense and rough*.
2. **Robert Moses** was involved with the Sivananda Yoga Vedanta organisation and worked closely with guru Vishnudevananda for over 20 years. He now lives in New Hampshire, USA, with his wife and three children. He teaches worldwide and co-publishes the journal **Namarupa** with Eddie Stern. All his family help to produce it. The course I attended was organised by Swami Govindananda of Sivananda Yoga Vidya Peetham.
3. Lord Ganesha is the Hindu God with an elephant's head and characteristics. He is the remover of obstacles and boundaries. When an elephant comes towards you, you get out of the way. If you know the Ganesha Dhyanam chant, you can sing it when you tap your temples in **2** on the opposite page. He is also known as Lord Ganapati. **Ga** represents **Intelligence**, **Na** represents **Wisdom** and **Pathy** represents **Master** - so meaning Master of Wisdom and Intelligence.

## Some accounts of first hand experiences of Thoppukaranam from my pupils

I have two pupils whose families moved from India to Kenya when they were young children. Both were taught the practice at school and it was usually used as a punishment.

An Indian pupil was taught the practice by her mother at the age of 5. She has done it every day since then, usually first thing in the morning and between 3 and 19 times. She is now 62. It was practised in her schools, both in India and Sri Lanka, mostly to improve behaviour and as a punishment. She does a variation, going up on her toes with her knees out to the side.

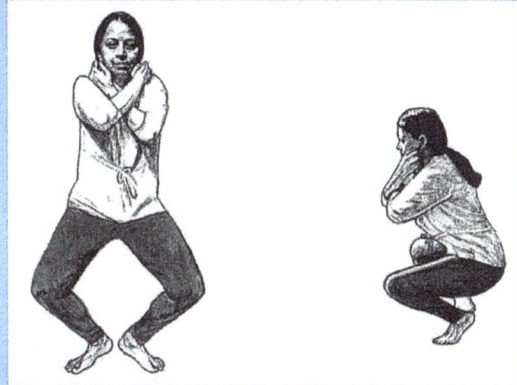

I teach a Malaysian family privately and the daughter (she is modelling this section) says her grandmother practises it daily and also does a tapping routine similar to the ones in the second section of the **Warm Ups**.

A pupil whose parents were brought up in Pakistan says they practise it daily. They all do a routine at sunrise and sunset which includes tapping and brushing off and is also very similar to the second section of the **Warm Ups**.

## Prelude to Thoppukaranam

**1**. Preferably, practise in the early morning, facing the east (the sun). If this is not possible, adjust to your circumstances. If you have been sitting in meditation or lying down, slowly come to standing.
Pause while bending forwards.
Take 5 deep breaths.

**Observation**: My pupil has long legs and can only bend down this far, as in **A**. I have tweaked **B** to indicate how far down people with an average leg length would go. This is an example of how body types must be taken into account when considering the alignment and appearance of the postures.

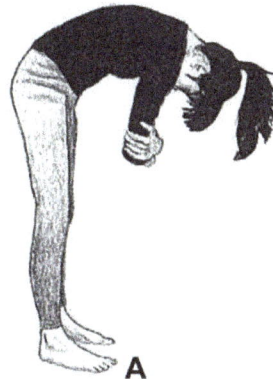

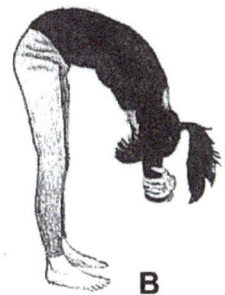

**2**. Slowly bring your head up. Tap the **Temple** area gently with your knuckles at least 30 times. You can tap above and behind the ears and the front of the head.

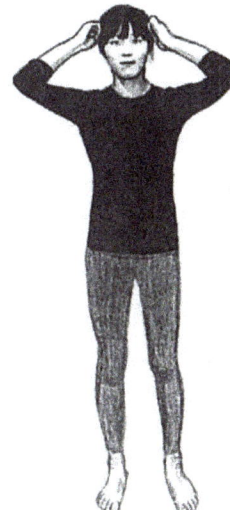

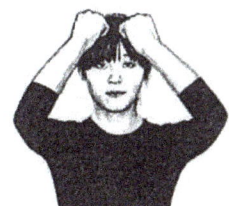

The word **Temple/Temporal** comes from the Latin word *tempus*, meaning *time*. It is used here because the hair of the head in this area is the first hair to turn grey during the aging process. *Information and diagrams by courtesy of Wikipedia.*

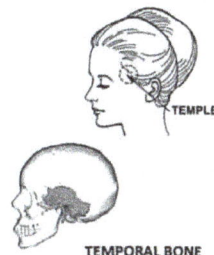

TEMPLE

TEMPORAL BONE

# Thoppukaranam or Super Brain Yoga

**1.** Place your left hand on your right ear lobe. The thumb is on the front of the lobe with the fingernail facing outwards, and the index finger is behind the ear lobe.

When you hold the right ear lobe in this manner, you energize and activate the **left brain** and **pituitary gland**[1].

**2.** Place your right hand on the left ear lobe in the same way, thumb on the front and index finger on the back. Holding the left ear lobe in this way energizes and activates the **right brain** and the **pineal gland**[2].

**3.** Maintain pressure on the ear lobes as you:
INHALE through the nose and squat down fully, keeping your back straight.
EXHALE through your nose as you come up.

Repeat this about 18 times to start of with and gradually increase this practise to about 10 – 15 minutes at your own pace over time.

**IN** . . . . . . . . **OUT**

1. **Pituitary Gland**   It is the main endocrine gland, a pea sized structure that produces hormones that control other glands and many body functions including growth.
2. **Pineal Gland**   Sometimes called the *Third Eye*; it is about the size of a grain of rice. It secretes Melatonin which helps to regulate the body's internal clock.

## Variations/Versions

There are many videos about Superbrain Yoga (sometimes it is written as one word) on the internet. I have presented the basic version of the practice but many variations/versions have evolved. Here are some of them:

**Superbrain laughter** is taught at a school in Bangalore, India. The children laugh as they come up from the squat.

In his book, **Superbrain Yoga, Master Choa Kok Sui**[1] teaches the most popular version. This is going up on your toes with the knees out to the side, as demonstrated by my pupil on page **33**. He also recommends that **young** practitioners face the **east** and **older** practitioners face the **north**.

Placing the tongue on the roof of the mouth is another variation taught by Master Choa Kok Sui and others. **Dr Eric Robins** says in his video, **Super Brain Squats**, "*This stimulates the Hypothalamus*[2] *which is the main antenna for sensing our environment.*"

Some practitioners pause for three seconds after the **inhalation** while holding the squat. Nobody I came across mentions anything about left-handed practitioners. My left-handed pupils sometimes choose to change their hands over.

I sent Robert Moses my draft copy of **Warm Ups** and he replied that he now teaches a different version of **Thoppukaranam**. He said this is the way it was traditionally done in the Hindu Temples to salute Lord Ganesha. It involves crossing the right foot over the left foot.

**And finally**: During coronavirus lockdown, 2020, I spent too much time sitting while finishing off this book. To compensate, I added my mantra to this practice and used it for my morning meditation. I closed my eyes, slowed down my breathing and concentrated on the point between the eyebrows. I found it worked well with the Gayatri mantra.
I do four breaths per mantra (4 downs and ups per mantra). I chose the simplest variation on page 32. Counting spoilt the meditation. So I carried on for a comfortable duration. I find it a very good way to start off the day and it remains part of my daily meditation.

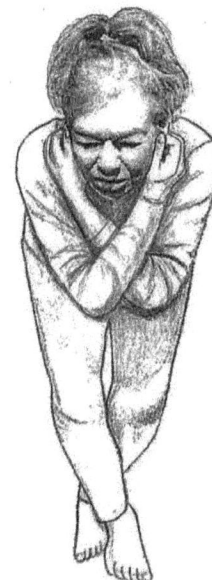

**Caution**: People fitted with a Pacemaker should avoid this practice.

1. **Superbrain Yoga** by **Master Choa Kok Sui**, 2005, is published by the Institute for Inner Studies Publishing Foundation, Inc. I can recommend this book to anybody who wants to learn more about Super Brain Yoga.
2. The **Hypothalamus** is the size of an almond and links the **nervous system** to the **endocrine system** via the **pituitary gland**. It produces the hormones **oxytocin** and **vasopressin**.
 I have come across several explanations for the practice of placing the tongue on the roof of the mouth. Some teachers say the tongue connects the **energy at the back of the body to the energy at the front of the body**. Others say it connects **the ancient part of the brain**, the Cerebellum, **to the modern part of the brain**, the Frontal Lobes.

# Sukshma Vyayama - Warm Ups

**Sukshma** means *fine and delicate* in Sanskrit. **Vyayama** means *to stretch and warm up.* In contrast, **Sthula** Vyayama means *dense and rough warm up.* These are ancient Indian practices.

In his book, **Health and Long Life[1]**, Swami Sivananda lists many types of massage techniques, including stroking (Effleurage), tapping, beating and pounding (deep tissue massage). Many schools of yoga still teach these practices but are not often found in the schools of yoga that are currently popular: They have been kept alive in systems such as Qigong.

Robert Moses looked at different warm-up systems and chose to adapt the one taught by Matt Pesendian called **Longevity Qigong[2]** for daily practice. The warm up system Robert taught is not identical to Matt Pesendian's warm up. I have drawn from both versions.

Maintain deep, rhythmic, soft Ujjayi[3] breathing throughout.

## 1. Focus the Mind

Stand with the feet a hip width apart. Place one hand on top of the other[4].
**Men**, left hand on the navel and right hand on top.
**Women**, right hand on the navel and left hand on top. Take a few deep breaths as you focus your mind and enjoy a moment of stillness.

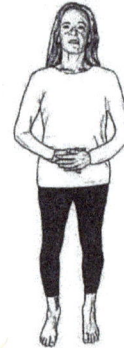

## 2. Gathering Prana[5]

**INHALE** as you sweep the arms out and up till the palms touch above your head. Look up at your hands.

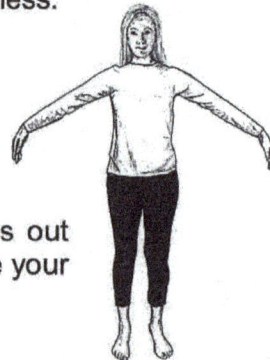

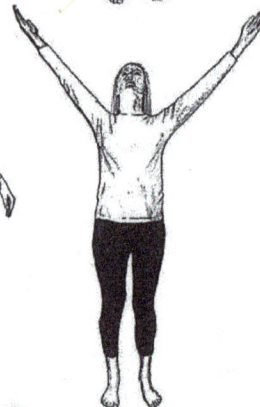

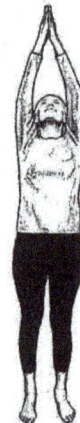

**EXHALE** as you bring the tips of the middle fingers together and slowly lower the hands. The palms are facing downwards. Follow the hands with your eyes until the head is level.

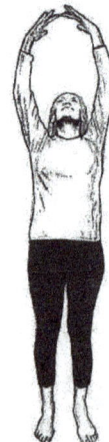

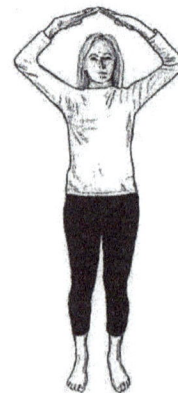

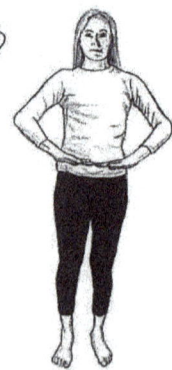

Take long deep breaths. **x3**

1. This was published by Sivananda Publication League, Ananda Kutir, Rishikesh, 1945
2. Please see www.mattpesendian.com/longevity-qigong/
3. See page 23
4. I asked Robert Moses if this was really necessary. He said it went back to ancient times and was very necessary. I take the middle road. Some readers will find this offensive and will want to disregard it.
5. **Prana** is the universal sea of energy that infuses all matter. In different traditions it is called **Chi, Ki,** and **Qui** and in Star Wars films, the **Life Force.**

## 3. Ankle rotations

Keep the feet a hip width apart. Move the foot you are starting with[4] behind and roll onto the tops of your toes. **Men** start with the left foot. **Women** start with the right foot. Rotate the ankles 10 times in each direction. Some people will get more out of the practice if they hold on to something.

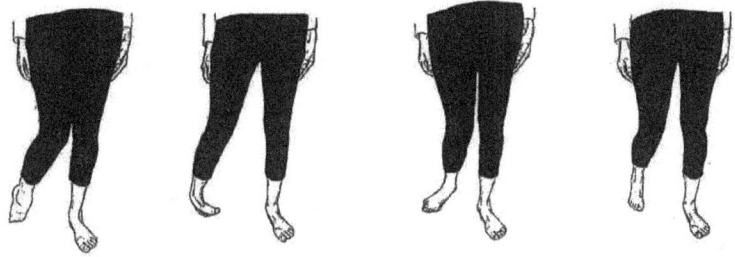

## 4. Meridian tapping[6].

This is in five sections. **A - Front and Back; B - Up and Down; C - Around the waist D - The groin and the glutes; and, E - Up and down the legs.**

## A. Front and Back

Stand with the feet a hip width apart and parallel to each other. Make fists with your hands and swing them from side to side with one hand on the front and one on the back. At each location tap gently 10–12 times. Synchronize your movements with soft, deep rhythmic Ujjayi breathing.

Swing your arms front and back. One fist taps the lower abdomen and the other taps the lower back

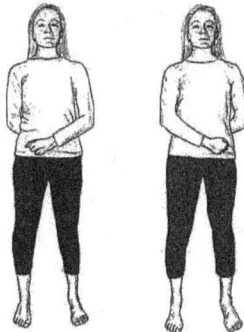

Move up to the mid-section, tapping around the waist.

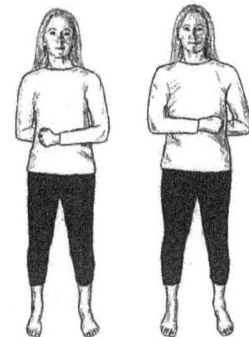

Move up to the chest and shoulders. Continue tapping.

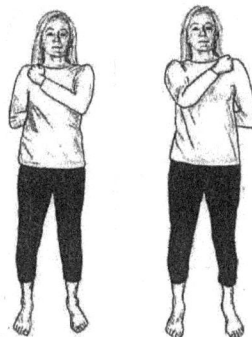

Move back down to the mid-section.                    Finish at the lower back and abdomen

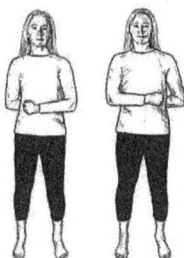

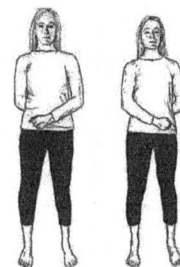

6. **Meridians** are 'energy highways' in the human body. Energy flows through them accessing all parts of the body. They have no membranes and cannot be seen but they can be traced in little spiral granules of **Hyaluronic acid**, see page 19

## B. Up and Down

Let the knees be soft and slightly bent and tuck in the tail bone a little. Make a gentle fist with your right hand. Tap each area about 10 times.

**1. Tap the lower abdomen.** As you move upward over the abdomen, straighten the legs.

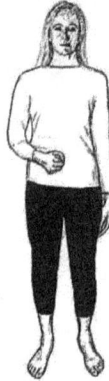

**2. Move up the middle of the chest**, tapping lightly, and towards the left shoulder.

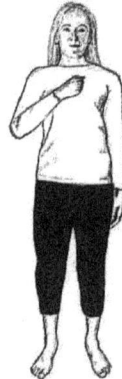

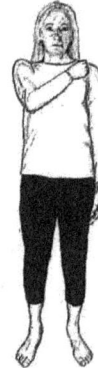

**3. Tap the underarm.**

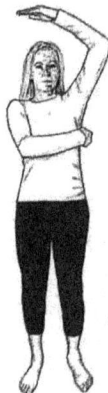

**4. Move down the side of the rib-cage.**

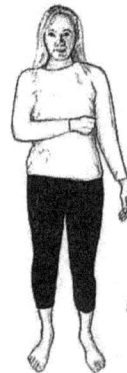

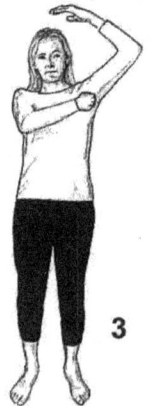

**5. Tap across the stomach, spleen and pancreas.**

**6. Tap up the chest** and across to the left again.

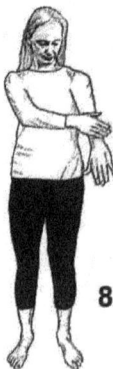

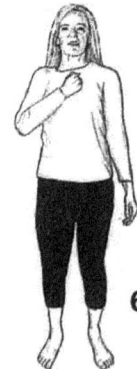

**7. Tap down the inner arm** with the palm facing forwards.

**8. Tap up the outer arm** with the right hand open and the palm facing backwards.

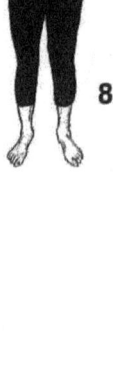

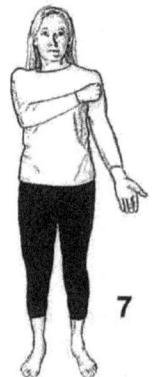

**9. Tap the side of the neck** with the open hand.

**10. Slide the hand down the outer arm** stroking and massaging.

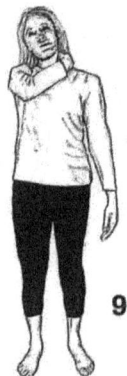

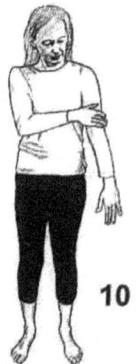

**11. Shake both arms out.**
*Repeat changing arms and sides.* I have reversed the images on the next page to help you remember the sequence

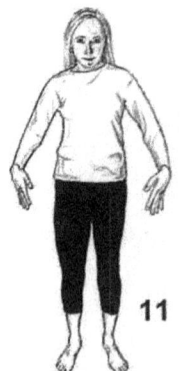

**Change to the left hand**. The only difference will be that you will tap across the liver and gall bladder instead of the stomach, spleen and pancreas.

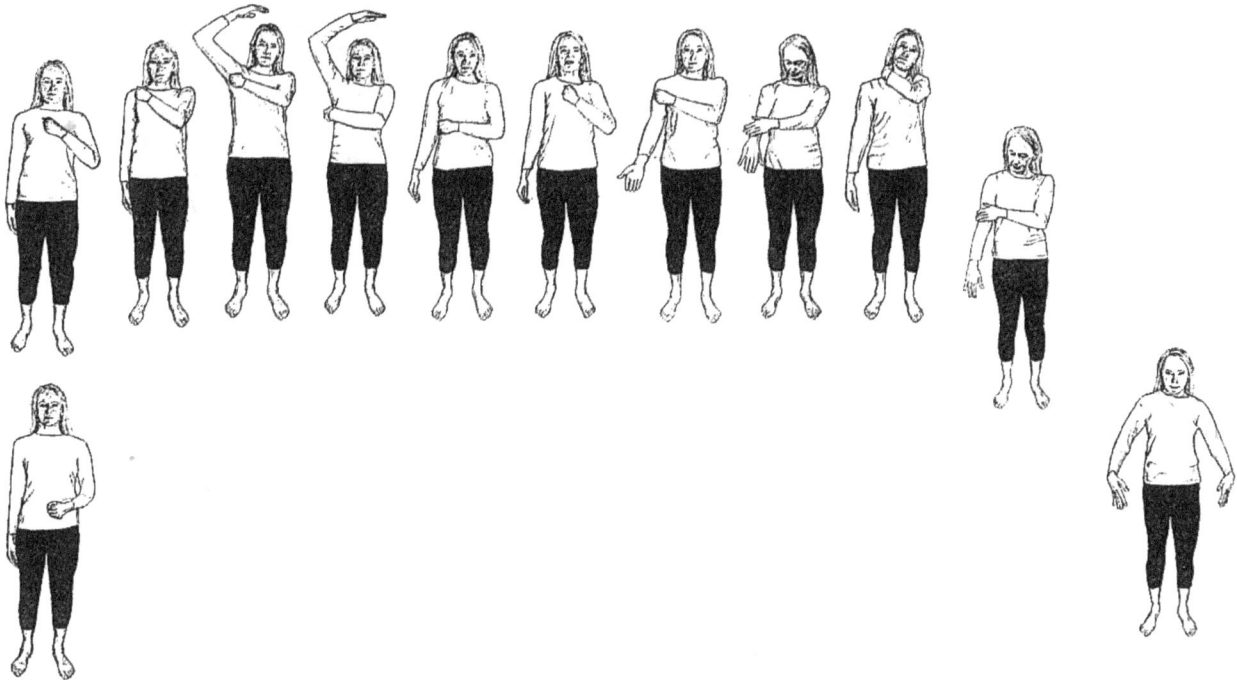

## C. Around the waist

Tap the waist with the sides of your hands. One of my pupils said she felt like a chicken.

Move to the back just below the waist and then to the kidneys, a bit higher up. Return to the sides of the waist.

Do this twice, tapping each area about 5 times. You can tap the back with the back of the hands or with lightly closed fists.

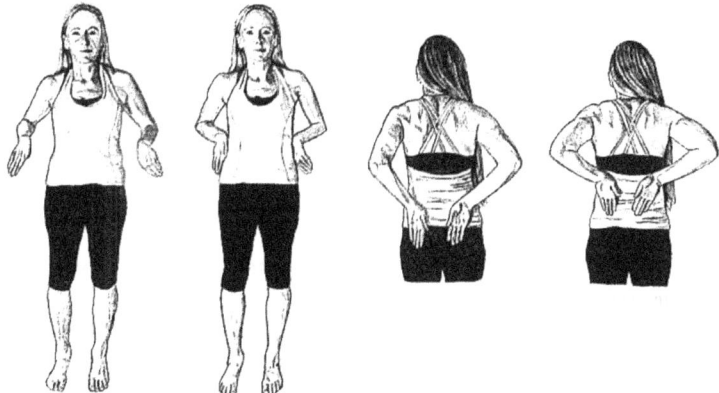

## D. The groin and glutes

Make the hands into gentle fists. Lightly tap the groins and then move round to the glutes.

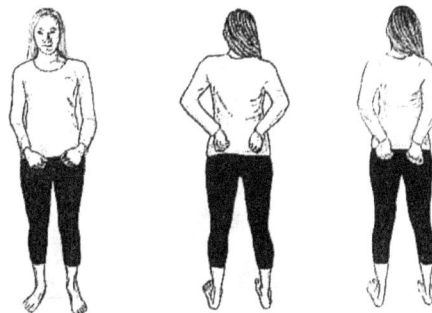

## E. Up and down the legs
Tap down the outer legs line.

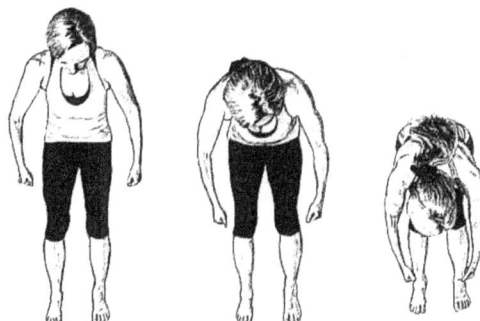

**Tap up the inner leg line to the groins**.

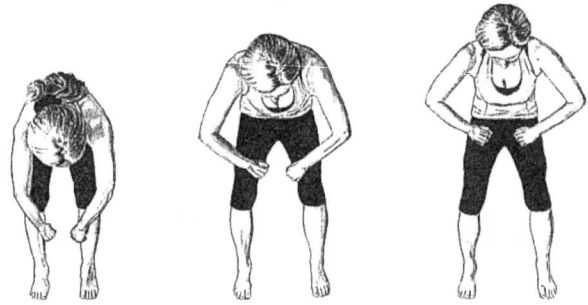

**Tap up and down the inner thigh**, between the groin and the knee. **x2**

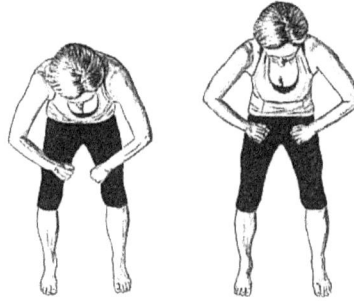

Return to the glutes and finish up at the groin.

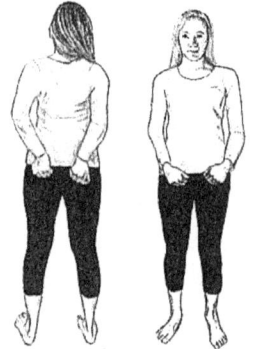

## 5. Neck rotations

Join the hands. Drop the chin and then rotate the head 10 times in each direction. Maintain awareness of your breath.

**Caution**. This may seem a bit more like **Sthula Vyayama**, a dense, rough warm up, for some people. If you have neck problems proceed with caution. Either leave it out or repeat only about 3 times on each side.

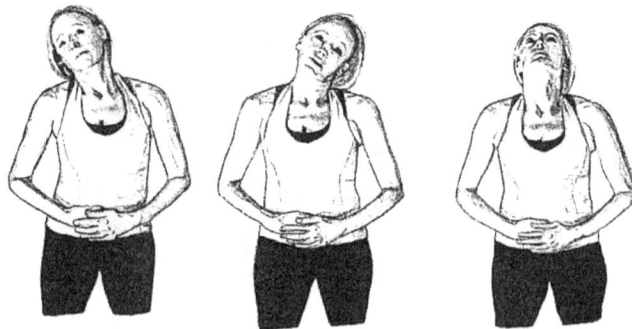

## 6. Shoulder rotations

Keep the arms relaxed by your sides and circle the shoulders forwards and backwards, 10 times in each direction.

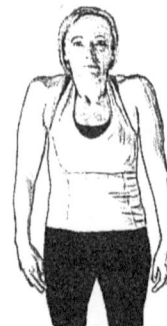

## 7. Wrist rotations

Stand with the hands in **Venus Lock** with the **palms facing downwards**. Stretch the hands above your head with the **palms facing upwards**. Lower the hands and press the palms together. Rotate the wrists 10 times in each direction.

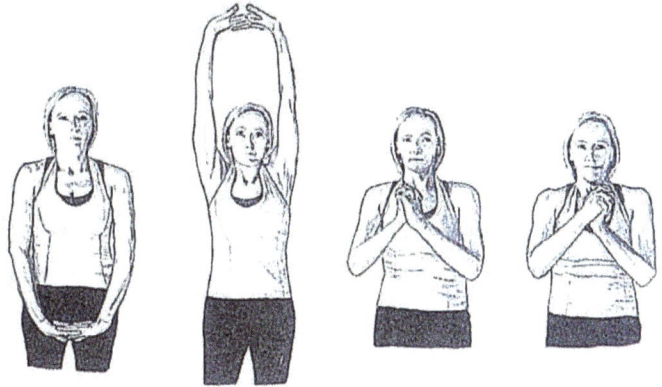

## 8. Gathering prana at mid-section

Hold the hands in front with the **palms facing upwards**. INHALE as you bring the hands to the waist and move the elbows out to the sides. EXHALE as you bend the wrists and move the fingers, first backwards and then forwards with the **palms facing downwards**, and stretch the hands out in front again. Repeat as many times as you want to.

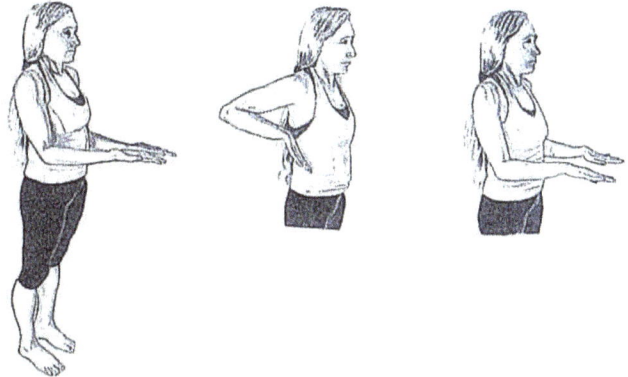

## 9. Circling the hips

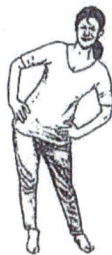

## 10. Circling the knees

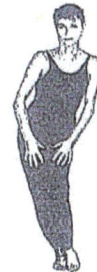

## 11. Eye and throat massage and brushing off the neck and torso

Stand with the feet a hip-width apart. **Rub the palms of your hands together** to generate warmth and energy.

Cover your eyes with the palms and hold for long enough to experience the warmth and vibrations.

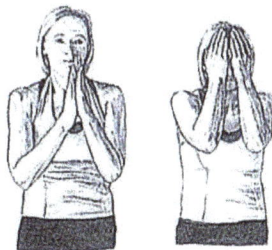

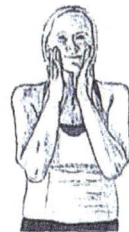

**Massage the jaw line**

**Lightly brush the neck and throat** (downwards).

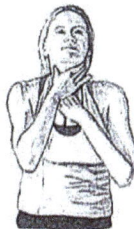

**Lightly brush the heart and abdomen.**

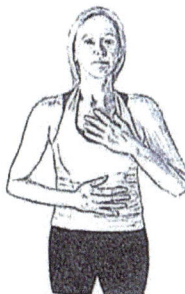

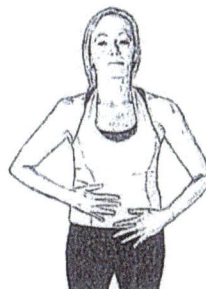

**Finally, brush off the torso.**

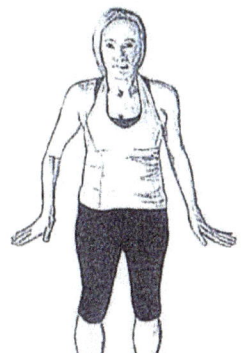

## Breath Counting on the Exhalation

I came across this breathing method in an article I had printed out from a very old Yoga magazine[1]. <u>Its strength is in its simplicity.</u>

**Inhale.** **Exhale slowly** and at the end of the exhalation, count the breath. Start with **1** and work up to **10**, i.e. ten breaths, and repeat it as many times as you want to.

I tried it in class, during the final relaxation, with pupils lying on their backs. I added my own suggestions: Intoning (thinking) the mantra Aum/Om on the **inhalation** and **exhalation** and counting in a pause at the end of the exhalation.

We were all surprised by the depth of relaxation we achieved. Obviously, you would have to use the deep breathing method of the **Full Yogic Breath** on page **6**. If you were using shallow, upper chest breathing, with minimal movement of the rib cage, you would not feel the benefits.

Since then, I have found different ways of involving this simple but powerful method.

**1.** It has evolved to be part of my daily mediation. I use half of my mantra on the inhalation and the other half on the exhalation and then count in a pause. I find it stops my mind from wandering.

**2.** You can add pressing pairs of fingers together, as described in **Five Finger Breathing** on page **19**. I press thumbs and index fingers together for the first five breaths and thumbs and middle fingers together for the next five breaths (**6 - 10**). I do another ten breaths, moving on to the ring and little fingers. You can repeat it as many times as you want to.

**3.** I find a simple version, without involving the fingers, by far the best way to get off to sleep when I'm having a restless night. It also helps to control unwanted, intrusive thoughts.

You can improvise your own ways of involving this counting method.

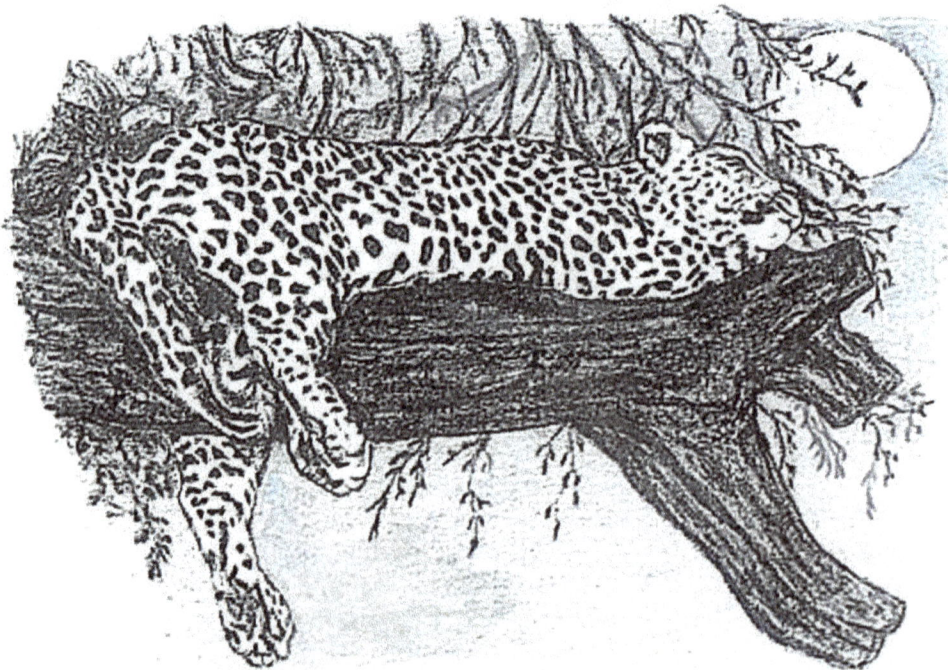

---

1. I can't date or name the magazine, but it is titled **'Meditating on the Breath'** and is written by **James Hewitt**.

# Introduction to Earth Flow

### How the sequence developed

**Tasha** contacted me about six years ago to say how much she liked my books. We met up at the Yoga Show in London and have had a catalytic yoga relationship ever since. She is modelling this sequence. At one off her inspiring Glastonbury Yoga Retreats she taught the last six postures of the sequence and the **Cleopatra** pose, **8**.

We met up to take photos for the sequence and she added a few more. To find out more about her, go to www.tranquillityinthecity.com

### Sources of the postures

**2** to **4** come from Robert Moses (see page **30**). **8**, **11**, **23 - 25** and **29 - 34** come from Tasha. **15** comes from the book *A Journey into Yin Yoga* by Travis Eliot published by Human Kinetics. **16** comes from one of Micheline Berry's *Liquid Asana* DVDs. **19** comes from Paul and Suzee Grilley's DVD *Yin Yoga: The Foundation of a Quiet Practice*. **25** and **26** come from Eric Schiffman, a US based yoga teacher. All the other postures come from general yogic repertoire.

### Cautions

Please observe the **Cautions** that go with **Bridge and Boat**, **9**, and **The Cactus Twist**, **20**.

### Additional notes

The transitions from **7-8**, into the **Cleopatra** pose, and from **11-12**, into **Animal Relaxation** pose, need to be practised carefully and systematically. It would be beneficial to practise these before working through the whole sequence. Avoid lowering the upper leg and foot to the floor too quickly in both transitions. I like to lower the top knee to the bottom knee first between **11** and **12**. Experiment with ways of pushing yourself up into the new postures.

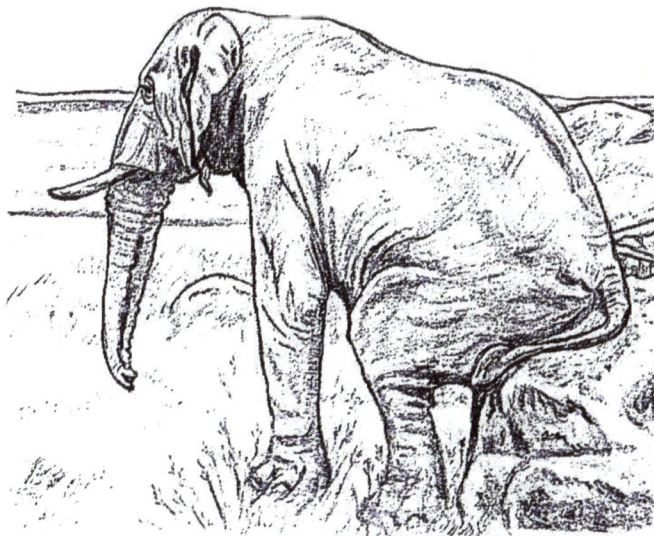

**The Seated Elephant Pose**

# Earth Flow

**1.** Lie on your back with the feet together. Bring your awareness to the breath.

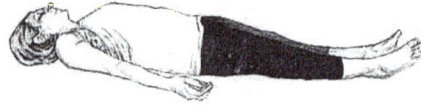

**2.** Move your hands out to the side at 180 degrees with the palms facing down. Bend the right knee and place the foot on the floor. **INHALE**

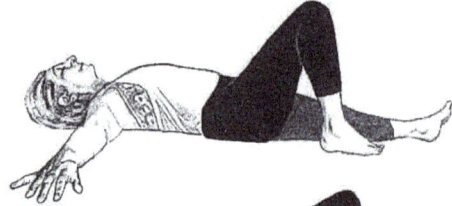

**3.** **EXHALE** as you push on your right foot and lift the right buttock off the floor. At the same time, rotate your palm upwards and look towards your hand. *Repeat three times.*
*Change sides and repeat.*

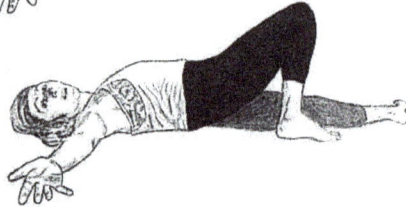

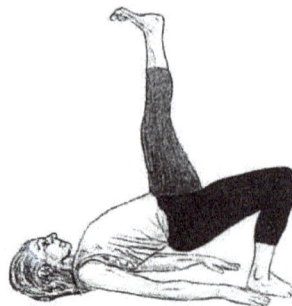

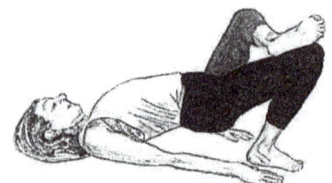

**4.** Wrap your left leg around your right knee. **INHALE** as you lift your right foot a short distance off the floor. **EXHALE** as you look to the left and move your knees to the right. Hold for a few breaths.
*Change sides and repeat.*

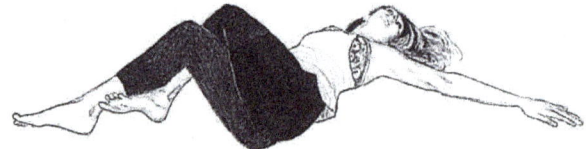

**Observation**
Some experimentation may be necessary. Some people feel a Piriformis[1]-type stretch on the side of the hip of the upper leg and others don't.

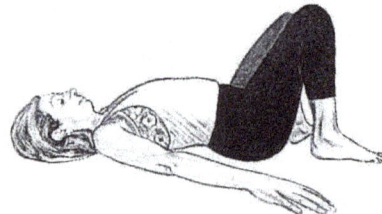

**5. Slow Bridge with Pelvic Tilt**
Bend the knees with the feet about 6 inches apart. **INHALE** as you tilt the tailbone downwards and feel the lower back arching off the floor, high enough to put your hand underneath. The hips will move forwards.
**EXHALE** as you tilt the tailbone upwards and feel the lower back pushing down into the floor. The hips will move back.

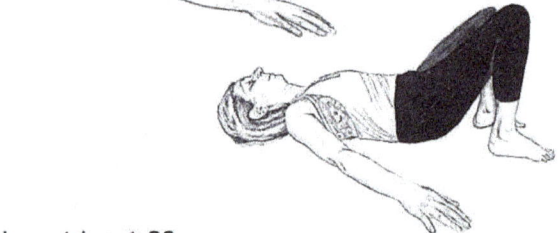

Now combine the **Pelvic Tilt** with the **Bridge** pose, taking at least 20 seconds to come up into the **Bridge** and the same time to lower down. The aim is to increase awareness of the spine. Try to be aware of each vertebra as you move very slowly.
Start by tilting the tail bone downwards and then slowly lower the spine to the floor. You will automatically pass through the upward tilt before you start to lift the spine off the floor. Push right up onto the shoulders and then reverse the movement, slowly lowering the spine and finishing up with the tail bone tilted downwards. *Repeat once or twice.*

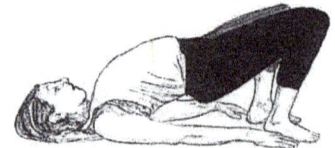

**6.** From **Bridge** pose, **INHALE** as you stretch your left foot up towards the ceiling. Push away with the heel.
**EXHALE** as you lower the side of the left foot to the right knee and push the hips up higher. *Repeat three times*, pushing the hips a little higher each time you lower the foot to the knee.
*Change sides and repeat.*

1. See Page **75**

**7**.  Stay in **Bridge** pose and push up on your toes, walking the feet a little closer to the hips. Stretch the hands behind you and interlock them in **Venus Lock**.  Push away with the palms.

**INHALE** as you lift the left leg.
Repeat the same procedure as in **6**, but this time, you will be pushing up on your toes.
From here, **don't change sides** as we are going to move into **Cleopatra** pose.

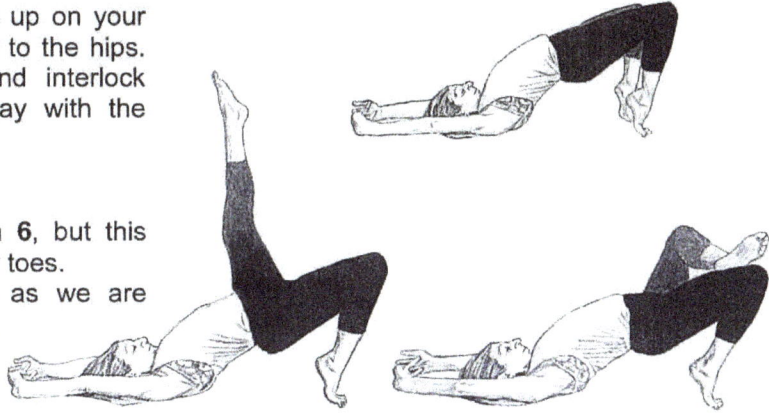

**8**.  Lower the hips to the floor, keeping the left foot on the knee.
Straighten the right leg and use your arms to push yourself to a sitting position. Move over on to your right side and rest on your right forearm with the hand out to the side.
  Slowly lower the left lower leg and knee to the floor on the right.  Place your left hand on your head and twist round looking up to the left in **Cleopatra** pose.
*Hold the pose* for as long as you comfortably can and experience the unusual stretch in the mid-section of your body.  Different body types will feel the stretch in different places.

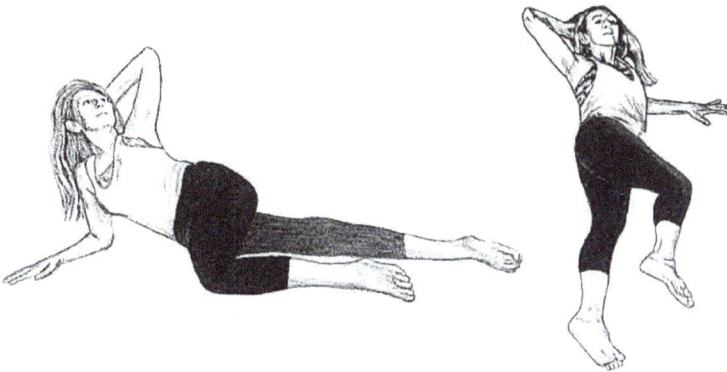

*Return to 7 .  Change sides and repeat*.

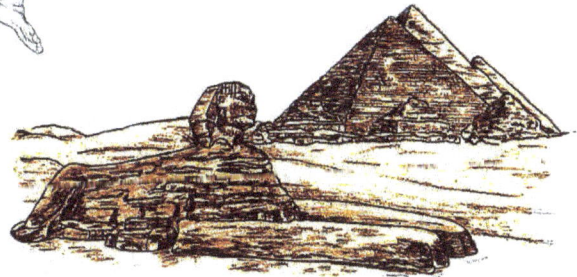

**9.  Bridge and Boat**

**INHALE** into **Bridge** pose with your hands behind your head.

**Caution**.  This is a demanding abdominal exercise.  If you have back problems, you may prefer to not to do it.

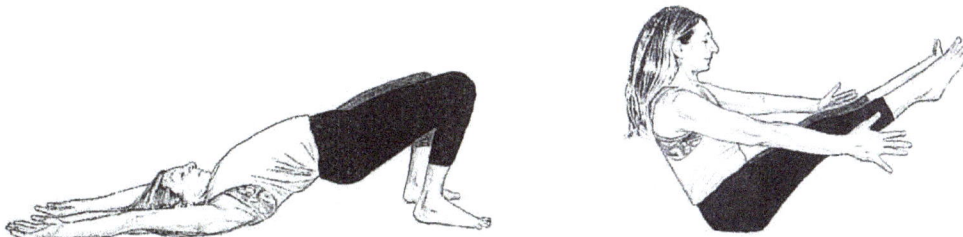

**EXHALE** into **Boat** pose, as illustrated.
*Repeat three times*.

After you have moved from **Bridge** to **Boat** three times in three breaths, you can adapt to a more leisurely pace and pause in the postures. It is quite sufficient to come into a low **Boat** with the feet and shoulders a short distance off the floor.
**For an easier version**, you can start with a **Half Boat**. Keep one foot on the floor or lift it slightly off the floor. You can also bend the knees if you find it too demanding.

### 10. Toe tapping with elbow and knee

Start on your back with both knees bent and the feet wide apart. Interlock your hands on the back of your head and lift the head and shoulders a little. Now lift the feet a little. This is your **mid-point**. **INHALE**.

**EXHALE** as you move your left elbow to your left knee and tap your right toes to the floor.

**INHALE** back to the **mid-point**, 10.
*Change sides and repeat*, bringing your right elbow to the right knee and tapping your left toes to the floor.
**Continue** for as long as you want to and then hold the twists to the side for longer if desired.

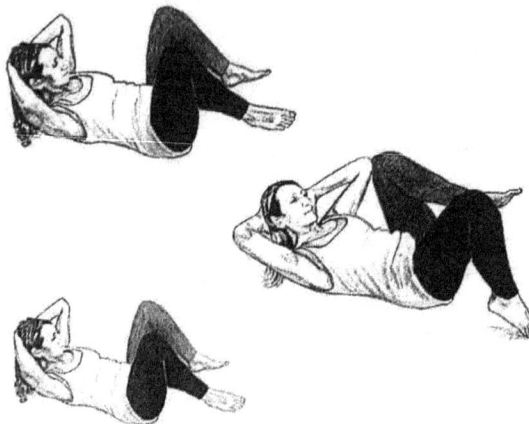

11. In preparation for **Animal Relaxation** pose, roll over onto your right side with your ear resting on the upper arm. Catch hold of your left foot with your left hand and slowly pull the knee back, stretching the front of the thigh.
Hold for as long as you want to, increasing the stretch on the **exhalations** and pushing the right fingers away from the toes.

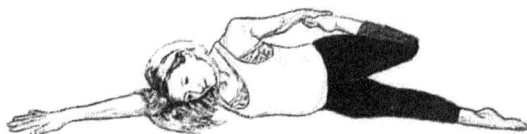

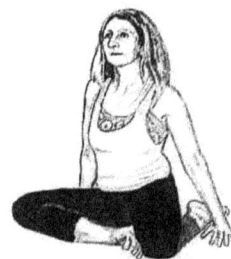

12. When you are ready, let go of the left foot. Bending your right knee a little, use your arms and hands to push yourself to sitting with your left foot still behind you. The right foot rests against the left inner thigh in **Animal Relaxation** pose.

13. Move the hands behind and push up on knuckles, fingertips or palms. As you lift the chest, the neck will move backwards in line with the spine and the chin will rise. **Hold for a few breaths** in **Backward Animal Relaxation** pose.

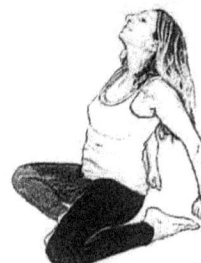

14. Slowly bring the head forwards and return to **12**. Rotate round to the right and lower down over the right thigh, coming into **Forward Animal Relaxation** pose. You can rest your forearms on the floor and make a pillow for your head with your hands or you can search for a comfortable alternative.

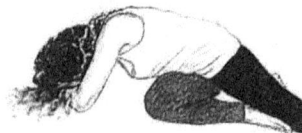

15. Straighten the right leg and slide your right hand along the inside of the leg. Catch hold of the heel or inner leg.
Bring your left hand over your head. Rotate the left shoulder back and look up to the left. **Hold for as long as you need to**.

When you are ready, come out of the posture carefully and return to **11**. *Change sides and repeat*.

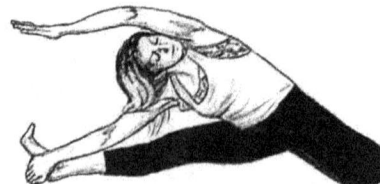

### 16. Side to Side Abs

Come to sitting with legs bent and the feet together. Interlock your hands behind your head and lift the feet a little, coming into your **mid-point**. Follow the breathing instructions for **10**.

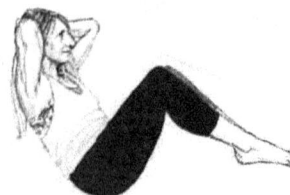

Straighten the right leg and place the back of your left arm/hand on the outside of the right leg.

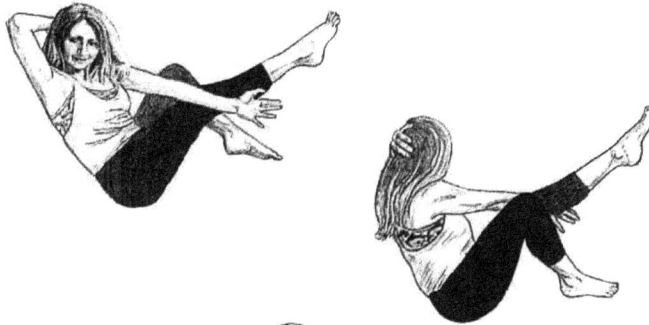

**Return to the mid-point**, **16**, and then change sides.

*Repeat as many times as you want to*.

### 17. Sitting Twists

Sit with your right leg straight and the left foot on the floor on the outside of your right leg.
 Depending on your arm/shoulder ratio, either catch hold of the left knee with your right hand or slide the right arm down the outside of the left leg.  Pull or push the left knee to the right and twist round to the left. You can improvise other variations
 Sit up straight with your left hand on the floor and hold for a few breaths as you twist round more to the left on the **exhalations**.

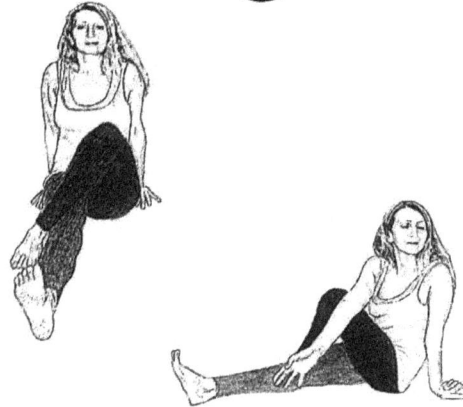

**18.** If you have broad shoulders and short arms you may have difficulty with this twist so don't feel discouraged if your arms won't cooperate.
  Move your left hand behind your back and the right hand back towards it under the left thigh.  **Bind** the fingers/hands together and *hold for a few breaths*.

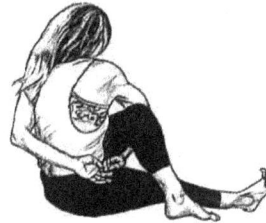

### 19. The Mongoose Twist

Keep your feet in the same position but twist round the other way, to the right, rolling onto your right hip.
  Place the heel of the left hand on the left knee with the fingers pointing upwards and push the left knee away.
  With your right hand supporting you, twist round to the right.

You will need to experiment to find the full potential of this ingenious twist. Your right arm can be bent or straight. Search till you find the best distance from your body for the right hand.
  You will know when you have found the correct positioning because you will feel an unusual, dynamic stretch from the top of the thighs, all the way along the abdomen and above.
*Hold for as long as you want to*.

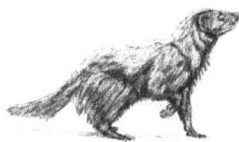

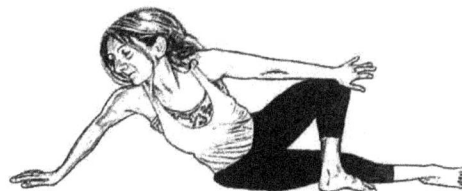

**Return to 17**. *Change sides and repeat*.

### 20. The Cactus Twist[1]

Sit with the feet about 6 inches (15 cm) apart and the knees slightly bent. Hold the hands up in **Cactus Arms**.

**Caution**. If you have back problems, limit the time you spend in the **backward** twist.

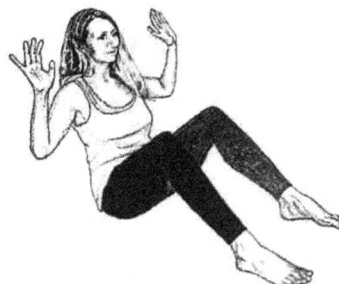

**1**.  The arms held in this way are sometimes called **Goddess Arms**, **Goalpost Arms** or **Cactus Arms**.  I have used **Cactus Arms** here because it is in the **Earth Flow Sequence**.

**21**.  Lean backwards and twist round to the right.

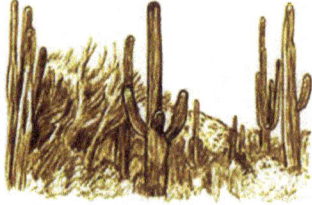

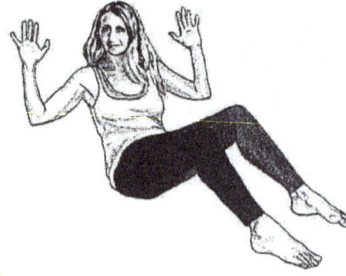

**22**.  While maintaining the backward tilt, place your right fingertips to the floor on the right side, away from the hips, and the left fingers on the left side towards the feet. *Hold for a few breaths.*
*Repeat as many times as you want to.*
**You may choose to rest between repetitions** by leaning forward with the elbows between the knees and holding the feet or inner legs.

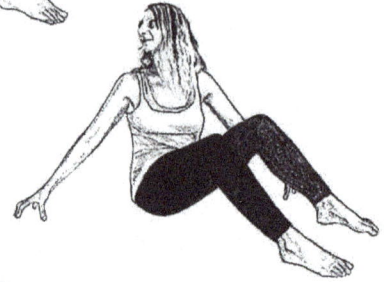

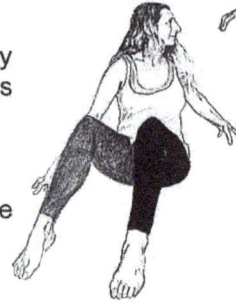

This illustration shows fingertips to the floor on the other side.

### 23.  Child's Pose Variations
Sink back into **Child's Pose** with the knees together and the arms along the sides of the legs.

**24**.  Bring your arms forwards with the palms together and the forearms resting on the floor.
 Separate the fingers and stretch the thumbs towards the ceiling.

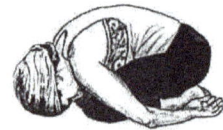

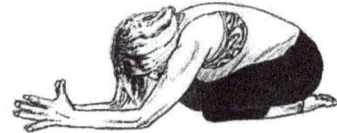

**25**.  **INHALE** as you swing forwards and rest with your thumbs in the space between the eyebrows.  If you have long thumb nails, rest them below the eyebrows.
**EXHALE** back to **24** and feel the stretch on the lower spine.  *Repeat three times at your own pace.*

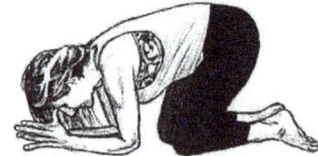

**26**.  Stretch the arms forward in **Extended Child's Pose**.  Widen the knees and bring the big toes together.  Push back with the hips.

**27**.  **INHALE** as you dig in with the fingertips and pull yourself forwards.
 **EXHALE** back into **26** and push back with the hips again.  *Repeat three times at your own pace.*

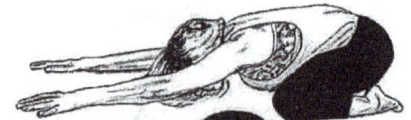

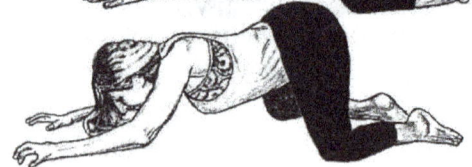

**28**.  Move into **Sphinx** pose.  The forearms are on the floor with the elbows rotated inwards. Start with the thighs, knees and ankles together.

### 29.  Swimming
Cross your left foot over your right foot.  **INHALE** as you lift your legs and bring your elbows back.  Hover there for a short while with the palms facing downwards.

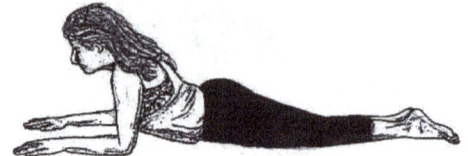

**30**.  **INHALE** as you bring the backs of your hands together and stretch the hands forwards.
**EXHALE** as you bring them back to **29**.
*Repeat as many times as you want to.*

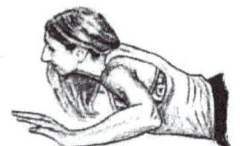

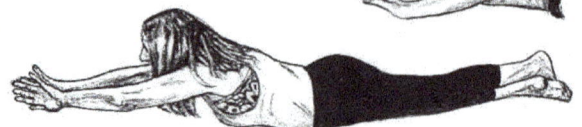

**31**. Lower down and rest if necessary before crossing the legs over the other way with the right foot on top.

Return to **29** and then imitate the **crawl** stroke. Stretch one hand forwards and the other back, coordinating the breath and keeping the arms and legs off the floor.

Continue for as long as you want to and then return to the **Sphinx** pose, **28**. Rest if necessary.

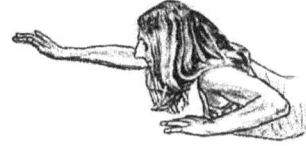

## 32. Sphinx Variations

Bend the left knee and lift the foot towards the ceiling. **INHALE** as you look over your right shoulder. Hold for a few breaths.

For a more dynamic stretch, lift your left knee a short distance off the floor, only an inch or two.
*Change sides when you are ready.*

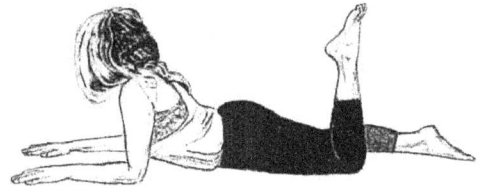

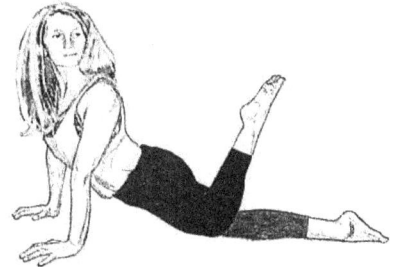

**33**. The next posture may need some experimentation to accommodate different body types.

Push up on your hands, lifting your abdomen off the floor. Bend the left knee and look over your left shoulder towards your foot. The knees stay on the floor and together unless you want to make it more demanding by lifting the left knee a little.
*Change sides when you are ready.*

**34**. Return to **Sphinx** pose, **28**.

Look over your left shoulder and push away with your right foot. The ankles may separate a little.

Hold for a few breaths, pushing away on the **exhalations**.
*Change sides and repeat a few times.*

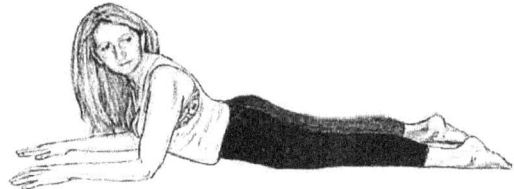

## 35. Back Breathing

Make a pillow with your hands and rest your forehead on them.
Bring your awareness to the breath. Feel the movement in your back when you breathe.

**A**. Concentrate for at least eight breaths on the movement of the **rib cage and upper back**. Try to feel as much expansion and contraction as you can in the rib cage[1]. Even breathe into the back and push the ribs apart, exaggerating it.

**B**. Move down to the **waist**. You should feel it expanding, back, sides and front, as you **breathe in** and the diaphragm moves down and out. It will contract as you **breathe out** and the diaphragm moves up into the rib cage again. See how much movement you can create around the waist if you move your diaphragm more.

**C**. Move down **below the waist**. There should still be expansion across the lower back and abdominal area when you **breathe in**. This is caused by the movement around the waist. See how much you can stretch across your lower back when you breathe. Even the Pelvic Floor expands just a tiny bit when we **inhale**.

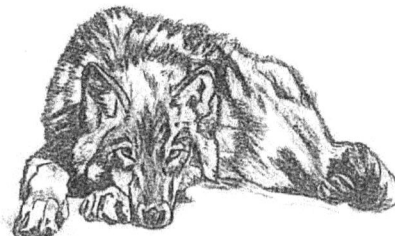

1. A pupil of mine in her forties said she didn't realise her rib cage could move.

# The Title of this Book

I liked the title, **Yoga without Boundaries**, and so did other people but it is ambiguous and needs to be clarified. The philosophers, **Aristotle**[1] and **Descartes**[2], have a great influence on the way we perceive the world. Both were **Dualists**. Looked at through their eyes, the world is full of boundaries. It was Descartes who concluded, *I think therefore I am*. If you reverse this to, *I don't think therefore I am*, you use more intuition and visualisation, and boundaries disappear.

This echoes the philosophy of **Vedanta** which has helped so many people. I write more about it on pages **63**, **73** and **93** . I had a muddled spiritual background. I was extremely religious and had a spontaneous Kundalini awakening (see Glossary) at about the age of 10. I was brought up Church of England but attended a Roman Catholic secondary school (St Joseph's Convent in Reading). There were nuns and I was a boarder there for at least a year. I knew the four gospels almost off by heart by the time I left school.

As I progressed through life, stopped going to church and read lots of books, I became confused. When I took my Yoga Teachers Training Course in my early 50's, I was taught the philosophy of Vedanta and it was like a light being switched on. Suddenly, everything made sense. I still love the Gospels, but I interpret them differently.

There are different schools of Vedanta, but the one taught by **Adi Shankara** in the eighth century has been the most influential. This is **Advaita Vedanta**. *Advaita* means *not two*. It is the concept of **non-duality**.

**Einstein's equation**[3], $E=MC^2$ resonated in a different way after I was taught Vedanta. I was amused to see a logo in the background of a video I watched recently. It was filmed at a **Science and Non-duality Conference**. The YouTube video is called **Non-duality and the Mystery of Consciousness** by **Peter Russell**. On the screen in the background, above the title of the conference was:

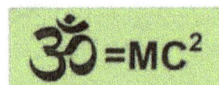

$$ॐ =MC^2$$

ॐ is the symbol for **Aum** or **Om**, shared by Indian religions/philosophies. It is generally thought of as the sound/vibration of the universe.

I have used the concept of Non-duality to make sense of the title of this book. Looked at through the eyes of **Advaita Vedanta**, there are no boundaries anywhere.

1. **Aristotle** was a Greek philosopher, 384 - 322 BC.
2. **René Descartes** was a French mathematician, scientist and philosopher, 1596 - 1650
3. **Albert Einstein**, German theoretical physicist, 1879 - 1955. The equation means **Energy = Matter**. **Deepak Chopra** takes it further and says,'There is no energy, only consciousness'.
#DeepakChopra #RajivMalhotra #MettaHuman

# Introduction to the Supple Body Sequence

When I need new ideas for my yoga classes, I often look through my many books for inspiration. I was not disappointed when I re-read **The Supple Body** by **Sara Black**[1]. It isn't a yoga book, although it incorporates many yoga poses, and the introduction has a section titled, **The Eastern aspects of modern exercise**. Similarly, I felt that some of the exercises in the book could be incorporated into a yoga class.

The postures used in this way are **1, 2, 3, 5, 13, 14, 16, 17** and **22**.

I have made changes, for example, in **3**, the **Swaying Angel** (I made the name up) the original version rests on the top of the back foot. My version goes up on the back toes. You can use either. I have also made suggestions to accommodate the average body, e.g., bending the arms in **16** and **17**.

Postures **7-10** and **18-20** are from general yogic repertoire. The interpretation of **18-20** is influenced by a sequence from **Yogaflows** by **Mohini Chatlani**[2]. I developed **11** as a way of transitioning from **10-12**. It makes an interesting **Yin** pose.

1. **The Supple Body** by **Sara Black**, 1995, published by Headline Book Publishing and Duncan Baird Publishers.
2. **Yogaflows** by **Mohini Chatlani**, 2002, published by Ted Smart.

# Supple Body Sequence

**1**. Stand with the feet together. INHALE the hands up with the palms facing and lean back a little, lifting the chest. Hold for three deep breaths.

**2**. INHALE the right leg up behind. Continue to breathe deeply as you stretch the hands up to the ceiling, without raising the shoulders.

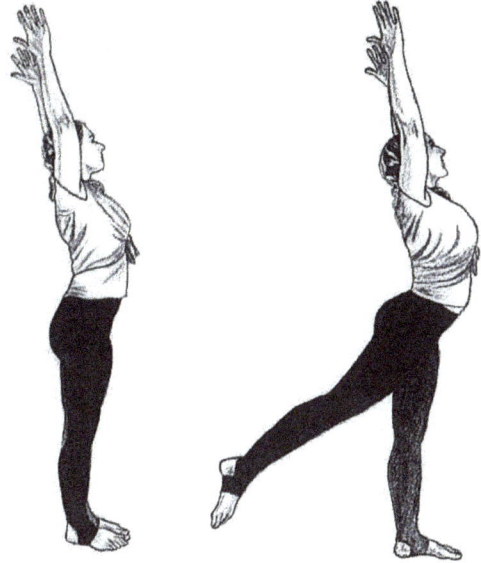

**3**. Lower the right leg behind to the left and push up on the toes. Lower the left arm and bend over to the left. The right arm curves above your head. Bend the knees a little, push down with the left hand and lean back slightly. Hold for a few breaths in the **Swaying Angel**.

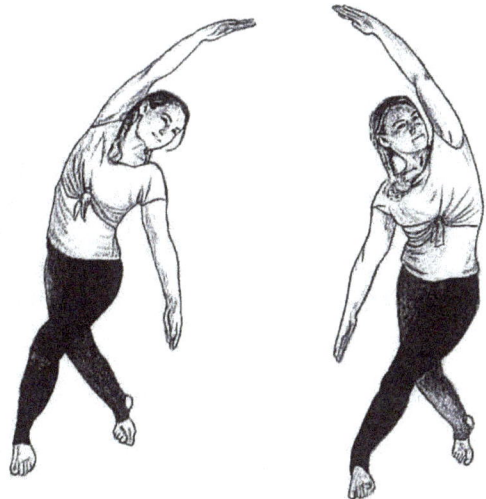

**4**. Keep the legs as they are but change the arms over. Now you are swaying in the other direction. Hold as you experience the subtle stretches in various parts of the body.
*Return to 1*. *Change sides and repeat*.

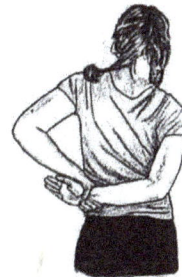

**5**. Bring the feet together. We are going to rest the legs while doing two shoulder stretches.
**Caution**. If you have troublesome shoulders, proceed with caution. Stop if there is any discomfort.

**A. Hand Cuff Stretch**
Bring your right hand behind your back. Catch hold of the right wrist with the left hand. Pull it over to the left, moving the right shoulder down and back. Slowly increase the stretch. *Change sides and repeat*.

**B. Scissors Stretch**
Bring your hands in front with the arms straight and the palms facing. Rest your right wrist on top of your left wrist. Every time you **exhale** move your right hand a little further to the left, stretching the right shoulder. When the time is right, *change the hands over and repeat*.
**For a variation**, you can change the angle of the stretch, e.g. point the fingers towards the floor or higher up. *Change sides and repeat*.

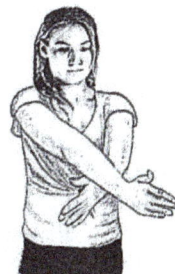

6. Repeat **2**, but this time, with the right leg forwards.

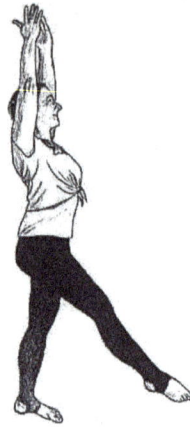

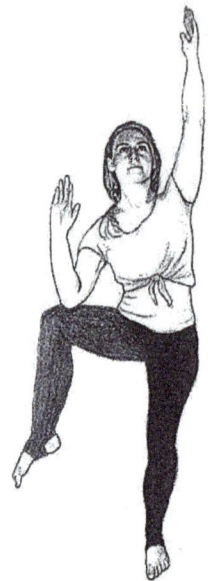

7. Swing your right knee up and out to the side. Rest your right elbow on the knee and stretch the left hand upwards. **7** and **8** are variations on the **Nataraja, Lord of the Dance** postures. Hold for a few breaths.

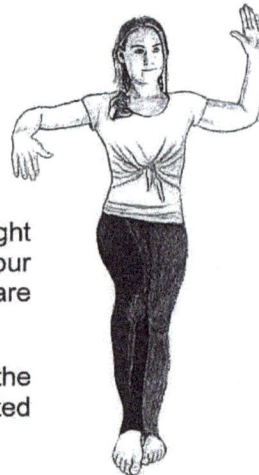

8. Bring both elbows to shoulder level and lower the right foot in front so that it hovers above the floor. Raise your left hand and lower your right hand so that the fingers are pointing in opposite directions.

The fingers pointing **upwards** signify **bravery** and the response to life's challenges. The fingers pointed **downwards** signify our **connection to Planet earth**.

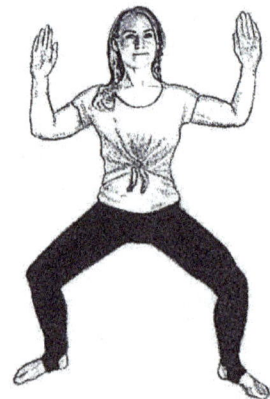

9. Step out wide to the right. Rotate the toes outwards and sink down into the **Goddess Squat**. INHALE the hands up coming into **Goddess Arms**. Hold for a few breaths.

10. You can choose which version you want to do next. All three have the tongue sticking out.
**A**. The **Lions Roar**, x3.

**B**. Look up into the top of the head but don't roar. This is the **Fierce Goddess**.
**C**. Look up and make a loud sigh in the **Sighing Goddess**. x3.

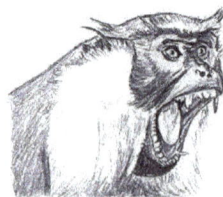

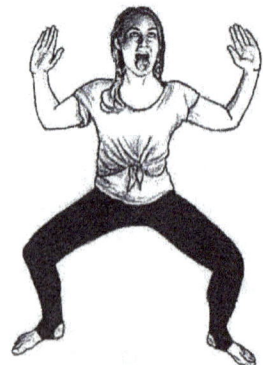

11. Lower your left knee to the floor while bending the right knee. Flatten the left foot. Stretch your right hand forwards and your left hand back, resting the fingertips on the floor. Move the hips backwards and feel the stretch at the top of the thighs. Hold in the **Monkey Pose**.

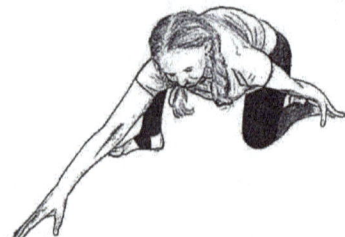

**12.** To transition into **Cobbler Pose** (also called **Butterfly Pose**), move your hands over to the left and lower the left hip to the floor, followed by the right hip. Bring the soles of the feet together and catch hold of the feet with your hands. INHALE the head up and EXHALE it down towards the feet, **x3**, while lowering the knees to the sides.

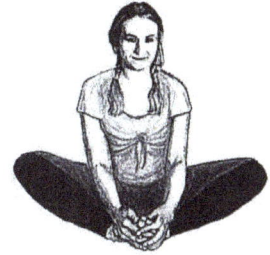

**13.** The **Rocking Cobbler**. While holding your feet securely, rock over to the left, bringing your head towards your knee. Then rock over to the right. The head remains forward throughout. Develop your own breathing pattern. You are likely to **exhale** as you rock down and **inhale** as you pass through the central position.

I find my pupils have their own particular way of rocking from side to side, depending on their body types. It becomes more enjoyable with practise.
*Return to 6. Change sides and repeat.*

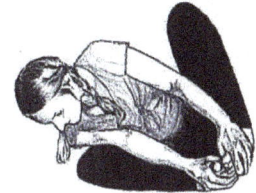

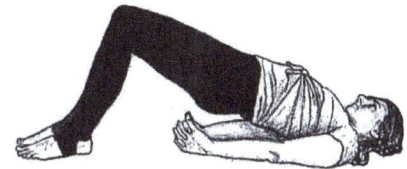

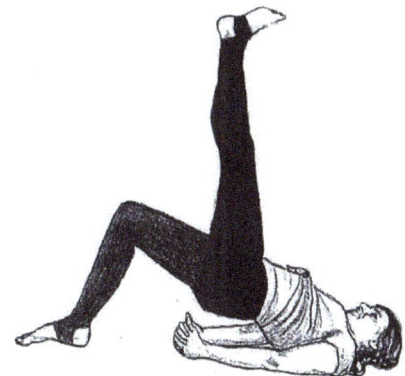

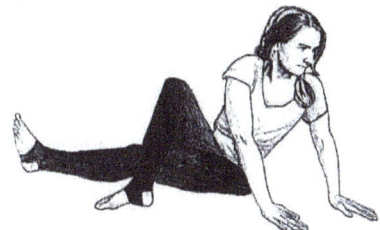

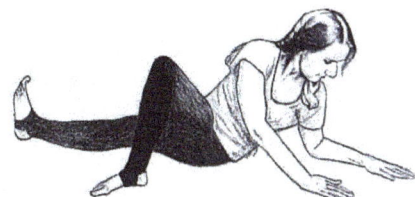

**14.** When you are ready, roll over onto your back and interlock the hands behind your head. With the feet together, roll over onto your left side. Lower your right elbow towards your left elbow. On the **exhalations**, push away with your right heel. Keep the foot on the floor and close to the left foot. To increase the stretch along the right side, tilt the hips forward a little. Hold for a few breaths in the **Elbows Together Twist**.
*Change sides and repeat as many times as you want to.*

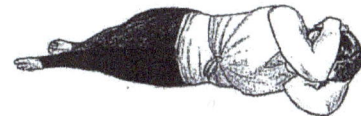

**15.** Roll over onto your back again. Bend the knees, with the feet under the knees and together. INHALE up into **Bridge Pose**. The hands can be interlocked, as illustrated, out to the sides with the palms facing downwards or supporting the waist. INHALE the left leg up and hold for a few breaths, pushing the sole of the foot upwards.

We are now going to make raising a leg in this posture a little more demanding. Lower the leg and hips and move your feet 6 inches (15.5 cm) forward. INHALE the left leg up again and hold as above. Lower the hips and rest if you need to.

If that was still within your comfort zone, move the feet another 6 inches forward and repeat. If you want to make it more demanding, repeat the procedure again.
*Change sides and repeat.*

**16.** Lower the hips and place the right foot on the outside of your left knee. Twist round to the left and place your hands on the floor. INHALE as you lift the straight left leg. EXHALE it down, **x3**. Lift it again and hold it there for a few breaths in the **Crossover Leg Lift**.

Some people will need to bend the elbows and lean forwards a little, as illustrated.
*Change sides and repeat.*

**17**. From **16**, after you have lowered the left leg, turn to the front and bend the right knee. Bring the foot close to the groin. Now slide the left foot in a semi-circle to the left so that you finish up with the leg bent and the foot behind in **Animal Relaxation** posture.

Place your hands on the floor, with your left hand close to the right knee, so that you are turning a little to the right. We are going to lift the bent left leg off the floor in the **Hip Lift**.

As in **16** you may need to lean forwards and bend the elbows. You can also widen the hands. As above, INHALE the leg up and EXHALE it down, x3, and then lift it again and hold it there for a few breaths. *Return to 6. Change sides and repeat.*

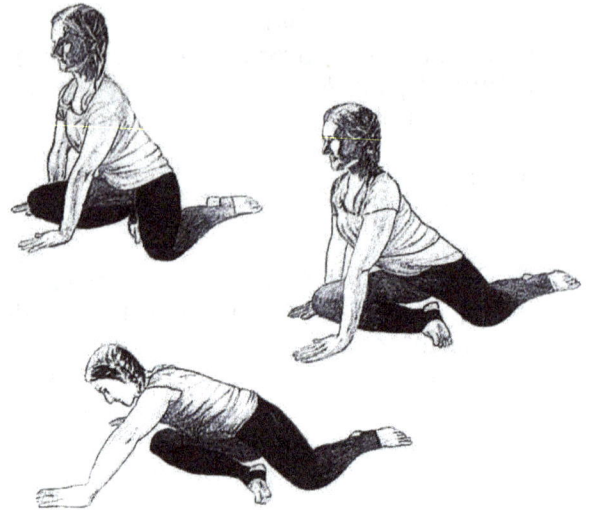

**18**. Come to sitting. Straighten the left leg and place the right foot on the inside of your left thigh, in **Half Butterfly Pose**. INHALE the hands up and EXHALE them forwards and down to the left leg or foot. Hold for a few breaths.

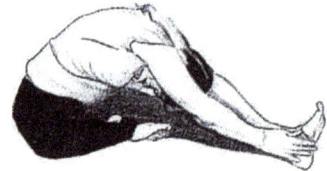

**19**. Lift your head and place the right hand behind you. Raise then hips and swing your left hand forwards and back. Stretch your left hand away from the left foot and hold in **Half Circle Pose**.

If you have a bad shoulder you can go down on the forearm instead.

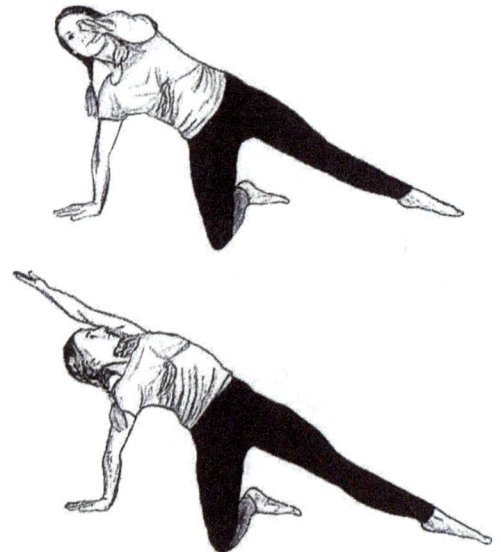

**20**. Wrap your left arm around your back and lift your left foot as high as you can (some people can lift it very high). Look down and hold in **Upward Half Circle Pose**.

Lower down and return to **18**. *Change sides and repeat.*

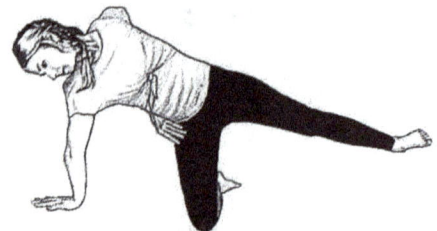

**21**. Roll over onto your front. Make a pillow with your hands and bring your awareness to the breath. *Rest for as long as you want to.*

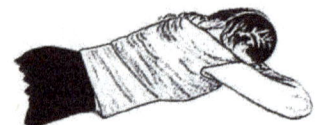

**22**. Move into **Plank pose**. Push up on your toes, with the feet together and the hands under the shoulders.

INHALE the right leg up, and EXHALE it over to the other side of your left foot, see below. Reverse the procedure so that your right foot goes back to where it was. **Change sides and repeat.**

**Continue** for as long as you want to. You can speed it up and **inhale** one way and **exhale** back the other way.

You may choose to go down on your forearms. The hips will probably rise higher if you do.

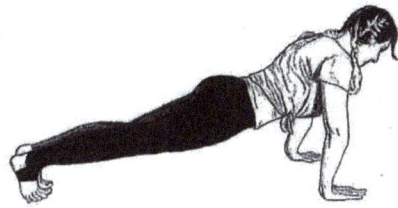

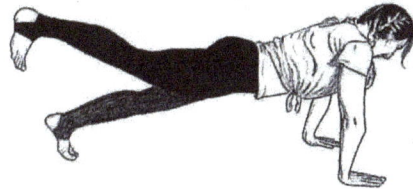

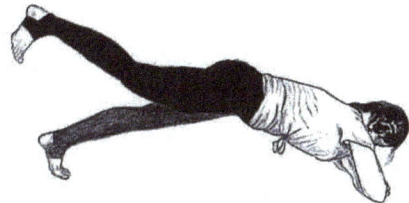

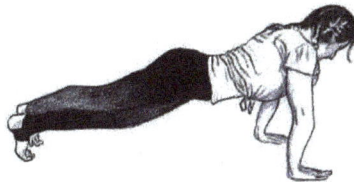

**23**. Lower onto the floor and stretch your hands out in front in **Ksepana Mudra (James Bond Mudra).** INHALE as you lift the arms and chest off the floor. Hold them there while you do one of these variations.

**A**. INHALE one leg up and EXHALE it down. Change legs and repeat as many times as you want to.

**B**. Lift the legs up and keep them both off the floor as you raise one and lower it. Continue as in **A**.

**C**. While keeping both legs off the floor, cross the feet over, change and repeat.

**Please note** that the distance people lift their legs off the floor will vary. Do not feel disheartened if you only lift your legs a short distance. It will still be beneficial.
You can bend your elbows and bring the hands back if you prefer, or put them on top of your head.
**Caution**. If you have back problems, proceed with caution and stop if there is any discomfort.

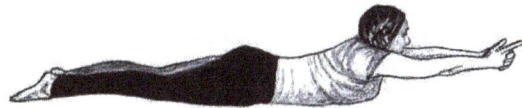

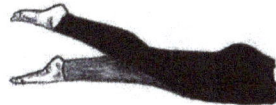

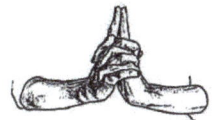

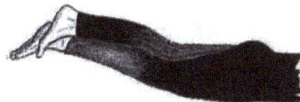

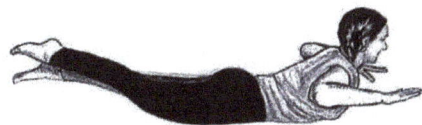

**24**. Swing back into **Extended Child's Pose**. The knees can be together or wide apart. Move the hips back and stretch the hands forwards.
**Alternatively**, rest in **Childs Pose** with your arms by your sides.
*Rest for as long as you want to.*

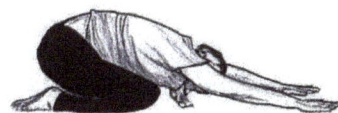

# Introduction to the Wall Flow

I developed this sequence after watching some online videos by **Erin Sampson** of **Five Parks Yoga**. I liked her ideas and found that some worked well when practised against a wall, e.g. **15 - 19**.

Using a wall for support helps you, not only to balance better and hold the postures for longer, but to align the postures more precisely. For example, in **11** and **18** the upper body can rotate in a more defined way. In **10**, **13**, **14** and **19**, the **Warrior** and **Triangle** poses, the support of the wall keeps the body in line and stops the head from moving forward. The security the wall offers can help us become more involved with the twists and stretches and the way we experience the breath as we hold them.

**Practical considerations**

Teachers will find that this sequence needs a lot of wall space. 'Heaven' is a flat wall with no obstructions. Those doing self-practice at home may be able to clear adequate space. Some yoga studios and village halls are fortunate enough to have uncluttered walls but when there are ledges, bars and radiators, some adjustments need to be made.

It is possible to make use of the obstructions by resting hands, feet and limbs on them or by holding on to them, so they need not detract from the enjoyment or functionality of the class. However, their stability should be tested first. Don't put pressure on anything that is not secured firmly to the wall. Although I have one pupil who likes doing **22** holding on to the sides of a radiator, I would be irresponsible if I advocated their use for this purpose.

If you are teaching a mixed ability class, the more advanced pupils could do the sequence free-standing if there is insufficient wall space. However, it would be best if they practised it against the wall first. They can then emulate the alignments it was possible to achieve while holding the postures against the wall. Alternatively, some pupils may prefer to practise this sequence away from the wall.

If you are teaching a large class, some pupils may choose to face in the other direction so they can see what others are doing. Teachers could then substitute **left** and **right** for **inner** and **outer**.

**Physical considerations**

**1. The inner foot position**. Position your inner foot carefully from **2** to **21** as it will be static apart from when you move to a 45 degree angle in **15** and change direction in **21**. It needs to be roughly 6 inches (15 cm) away from the wall and parallel to it. This won't be the right distance for everybody. If it doesn't suit your body type, experiment until you find the right distance for your foot. Your inside shoulder needs to feel comfortable resting on the wall.

**2. The Breath**. I have only mentioned the breath in **31**. That doesn't indicate lack of involvement with it in this sequence. Observe it as you flow from one posture to another, but when you hold the postures you will experience the breath in different parts of the body.

Someone new to yoga may not have learnt to relax the abdomen and expand and contract the ribcage when breathing. I find new pupils often have very limited movement of the ribcage. They should imagine breathing into the whole of the middle section of the body and feel expansion and contraction around the waist and movement in the back, above and below the waist. Those who are more familiar with yogic breathing will find the subtle changes in the breating experienced in the different postures interesting and engaging.

I have observed a disturbing tendency in some recently trained yoga teachers to instruct that pupils tense the abdomen in postures similar to those in this sequence. I have been taught that this has a negative effect on the **nervous system**. When the abdomen needs to tense and flatten it usually does it automatically. There is no need to tense the abdomen consciously in any part of this sequence.

## How to practise this sequence

This is a long sequence and it may take a long time to memorise. Once you are familiar with it, you can start to involve some elements of **Yin** and **Yang Yoga**[1].

**Paul Grilley** says, in his ground-breaking DVD, **Yin Yoga**:  *Yin Yoga is a form of Yoga that stretches and stimulates the connective tissue of the body.  It is intended to compliment Yang forms of yoga that stretch and strengthen the muscle tissues of the body. Yin and Yang are mutually beneficial and both should be practised.*

**For those who are unfamiliar with these types of practice**, postures are usually held for about 3 minutes in **Yin Yoga** (see foot note). However, consideration should always be given to levels of fitness and the demands of the postures.  I find it quite sufficient to hold some of the poses in this sequence for a minute and a half or two minutes.  Only hold them for longer if you are confident it is safe to do so.

It is not necessary to remain completely still when holding the postures.  Let your body yield to the posture and if you feel like moving part of the body to make it more comfortable, that is quite acceptable.  This is particularly relevant to the neck in this sequence.  If it starts to feel awkward and uncomfortable, i.e., when you are looking up to the side, move your head to a neutral position.

**When using elements of Yang Yoga**, flow slowly from one posture to another with full awareness. Find the maximum stretch or twist in each posture and then move on in a continuous flow.

## Variations

**1.** If you have knee problems and don't want to kneel on the floor, you can miss out **1** and go up on the outer toes from **2** to **5**.  Alternatively, you could place a chair against the wall and sit with the inner thigh on the front of the chair, as illustrated. You can stay there until **13** and either miss out **7** or use the chair for support in the **Standing Splits**.  Push the chair away when it is no longer needed.

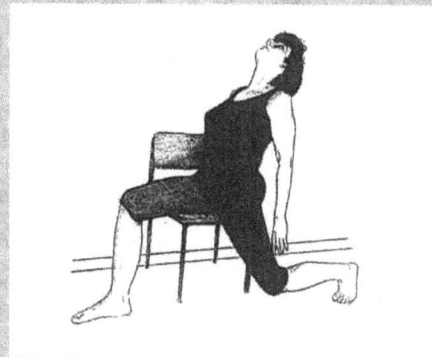

**2.** In **5**, you can mimic the twists in **21** and **22**.  You can rotate towards the wall, place your palms and forehead on it, then stretch away with the inner hand.

**3.** In **25** you can twist your outer shoulder back against the wall and improvise with the upper arm.

**4.** You can stay in the same direction after **30** but change the legs over. I have not included this in the sequence because it seems to have limited appeal and involves moving the inner foot.

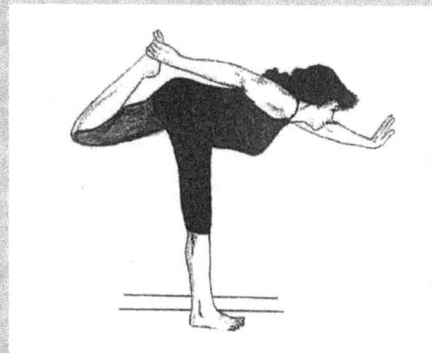

1.  Paulie Zink, a Chinese-influenced Martial Arts and Taoist Yoga teacher, introduced Yin Yoga to the West in the 1970s.  It was developed by Paul Grilley and Sarah Powers. It is a slow-paced, modern style of yoga. Beginners may hold the postures from 45 seconds to 2 minutes and more advanced practitioners may stay in one posture for 5 minutes or more.

# Wall Flow

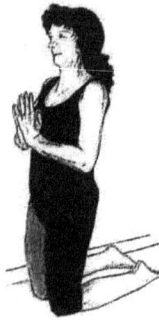

**1.** Kneel with your right knee about 6 inches (15 cm) away from the wall. Bring the hands into **Prayer**.

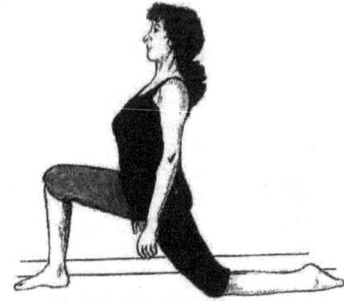

**2.** Move your right foot forwards so that there is maximum comfortable distance between the left knee and the right heel. The right foot should be parallel to the wall.

If you have knee problems, try variation **1**.

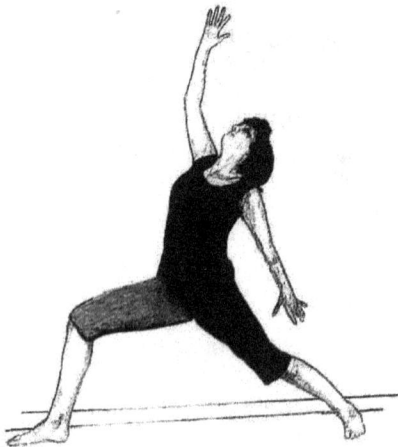

**11.** Bring the head up slowly and slide the back of the right arm down the inside of the right leg. Place the left hand on the hip and look up at the ceiling with the elbow, shoulders and head resting on the wall.

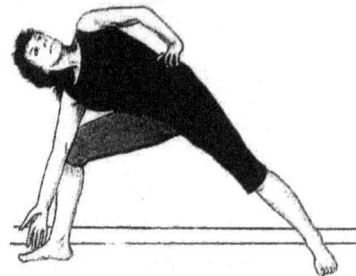

**10.** Move into supported **Backward Warrior**. Slide your left arm and both shoulders along the wall towards the left leg. The right arm floats upwards with the palm rotated forwards and the back of the hand on the wall.

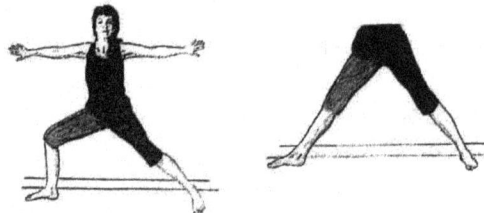

**12.** Return to **9** and then straighten the right leg in preparation for a supported **Triangle** pose.

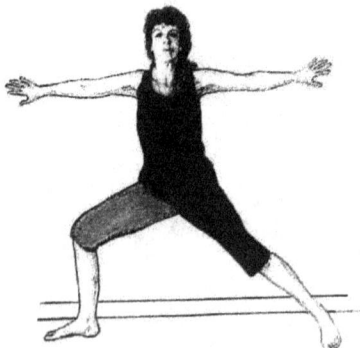

**9.** Move into a supported **Forward Facing Warrior**. Slide your head and shoulders up the wall and move the arms out to the side with the palms pressing into the wall. Lower the shoulders and push away with the fingers. Bring your awareness to the breath.

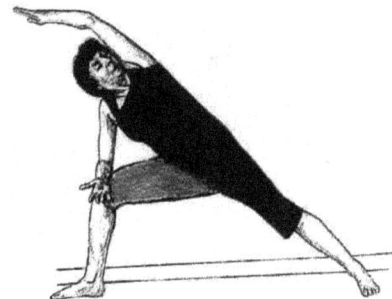

**8.** Lower the leg and bend the right knee again. You can move the left foot a little further away from the right foot. Place your right elbow on the knee with the palm facing upwards. Stretch the left arm over your head. Rotate the rib cage until your shoulders, head and upper arm are resting on the wall.

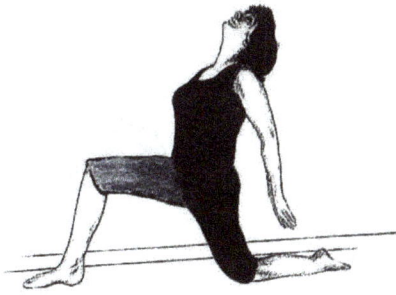

**3**. Swing your arms back in **Flying Bird**. Lift the chest and squeeze the shoulder blades together. Move your right knee forwards until you feel the stretch at the top of the thighs.

Look up and enjoy the stretch from the **Heart Centre** to the **Throat Centre**. The head will automatically move backwards but the neck will still be in line with the spine.

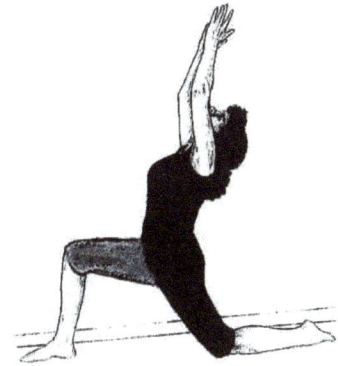

**4**. When you are ready, swing your arms forwards and back over your head with the palms facing, coming into **Crescent Moon** pose. Look up at your hands and lean further backwards if you are comfortable.

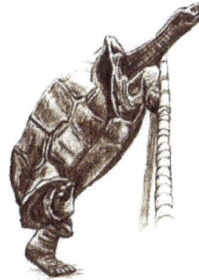

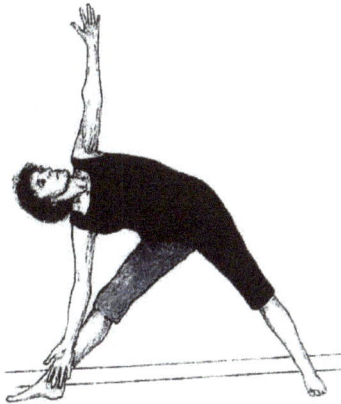

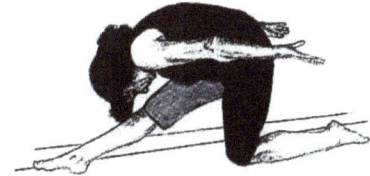

**5**. Swing your hips backwards and slowly lower your head, either towards the right knee or straight down. At the same time, bring your arms forwards then back into **Flying Bird** again. Sink the hips back as far as you can.

**13**. Rotate the palms to face forwards and, keeping your head and shoulders in contact with the wall, slide the back of your right arm down the inside of the right leg. The left arm will float upwards. Rest the back of the hand on the wall and push the hands away from each other.

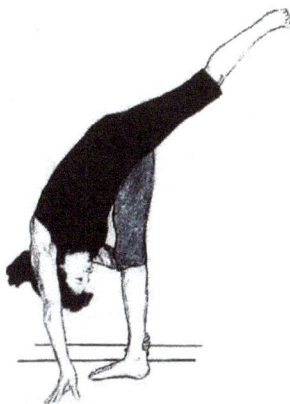

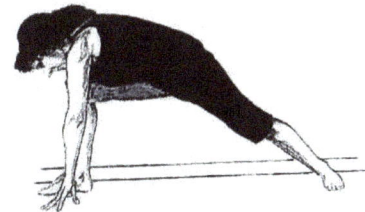

**6**. Swing forwards, bending the right knee and placing the hands on either side of the right foot. The back foot should be at a 45% angle.

**7**. Prepare for the **Standing Splits**. Push up on your left fingertips (you may prefer to rest your hand on a block) and lift the left leg as high as you can. The left foot and right arm rest on the wall. Catch hold of your right leg with your hand and encourage the head towards the knee.

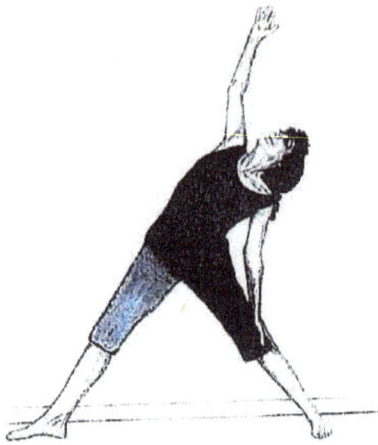

**14**. Slowly slide the head and shoulders up the wall and move into a supported **Backward Triangle**. Reverse the angle of the hands so that the left hand rests on the left leg. Look up at your right hand and feel the head and upper shoulder and arm resting on the wall.

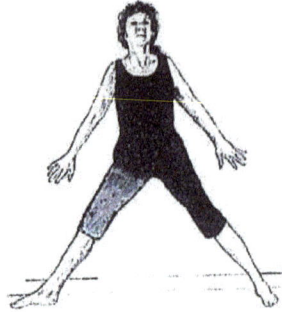

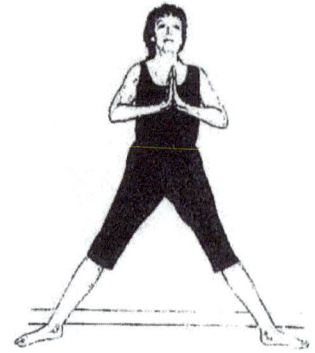

**15**. Slowly rotate to the left so that you are facing forwards with your upper body against the wall. You may need to experiment with the distance your feet are from the wall for these forward facing postures. The feet should be turned outwards and aligned carefully. Bring the hands into **Prayer**.

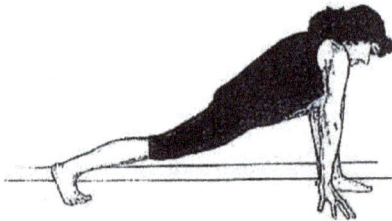

**23**. When you are ready, move out of the twist coming back to a neutral position. Lower the hands to the floor on either side of the left foot, in preparation for a supported **Upward Crescent Moon.**

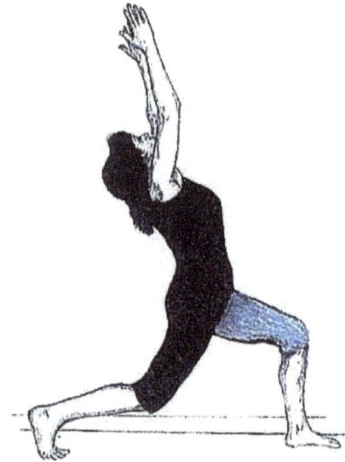

**24**. With the feet remaining in the same position, lift the head and the arms straight in front and then up and over the head. Look up at your hands and lean backwards as far as you comfortably can.

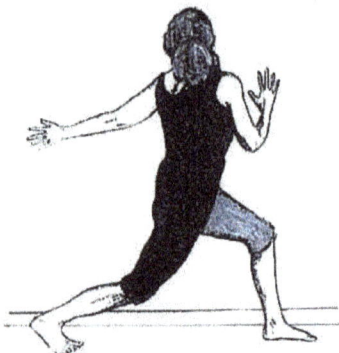

**22**. Keep your right palm where it is and stretch your left hand out to the side. Observe the sensations in your body and the breath as you slowly increase the twist of the upper body to the left.

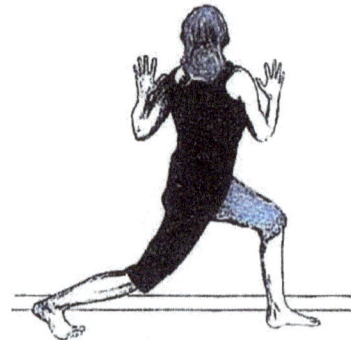

**21**. Lower the heels and rotate to the left. Bend the left knee and go up on the right toes. Twist to the left and place the palms of your hands on the wall. Sink down as low as you can. Your forehead can rest on the wall.

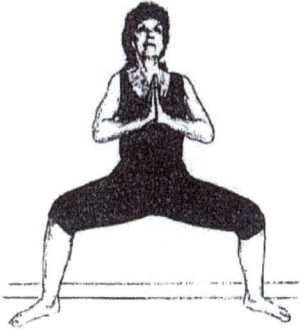

**16.** Bend the knees and slide your back and head down the wall, sinking down as low as you can.

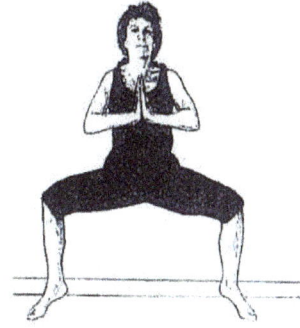

**17.** Go up on your toes and hold for a few breaths.

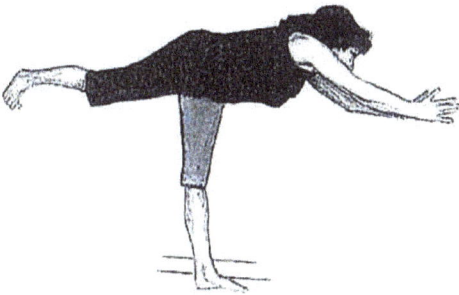

**18.** Lower the right heel and push up onto your left toes, lifting the heel as high as you can.

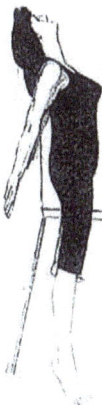

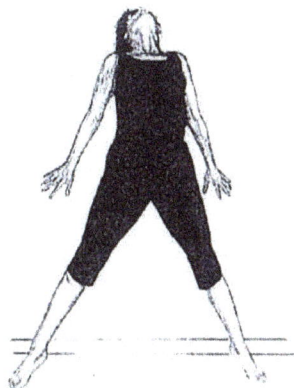

**25.** Prepare to move into a supported **Balancing Warrior** pose. Slowly bring the head and arms forward with the inner arm sliding along the wall. Look up as you lift the right leg and stretch the hands away in front.

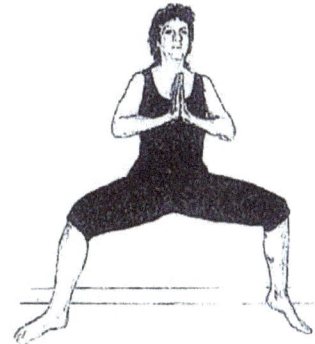

**19.** Change side, pushing up on the right toes. *Repeat 18 and 19 as many times as you want to.*

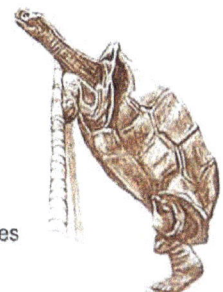

**20.** Push up on toes of both feet and slide your head and shoulders up the wall. Place your palms or finger tips on the wall. Lift the chest and look up at the ceiling. Lower the shoulders and hands. Hold for a few breaths.

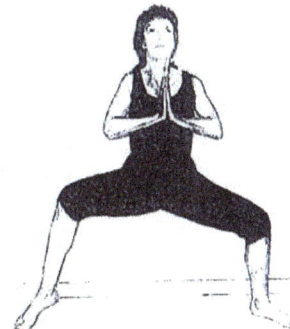

Even gaint tortoises do Yoga (joke).

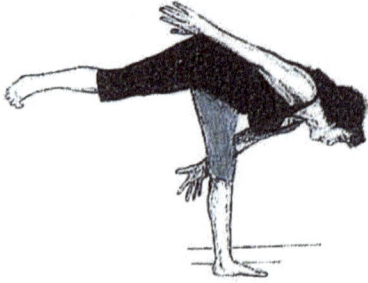

**26**. Swing your arms back in **Flying Bird**. Look down at the floor and lift your leg as high as you can. If the inner arm gets stuck there is no need to destabilise the body by wriggling it through. Let it stay there and lift the outer arm as high as you can.

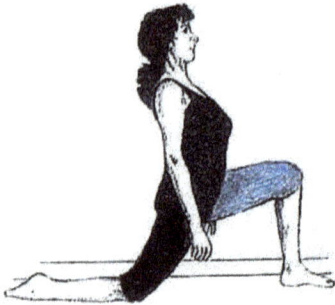

**27**. As you lift your head and swing your arms up to the ceiling, swing your right/outer leg forwards with the knee bent coming into **Standing Staff** pose.

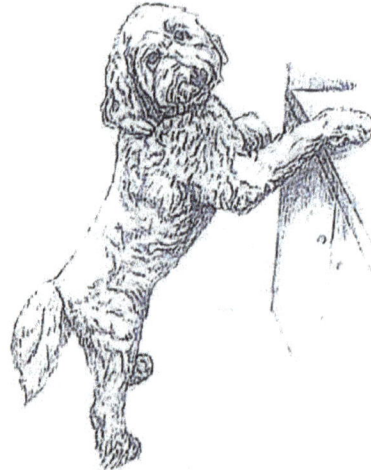

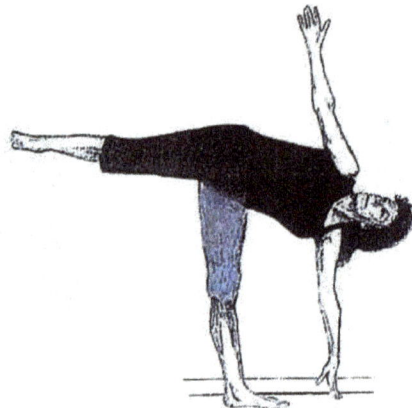

**34**. Lower the back knee to the floor returning to **2** but, this time, facing in the other direction. *You are now ready to repeat the sequence on the other side, leaving out 1 and proceeding to 3. You can return to 1 to conclude the whole sequence.*

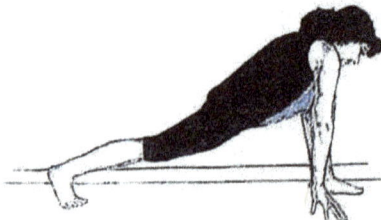

**33**. When you are ready, lower the right/outer foot to the floor. Bend the left/inner knee and twist round to the side, returning to **23**.

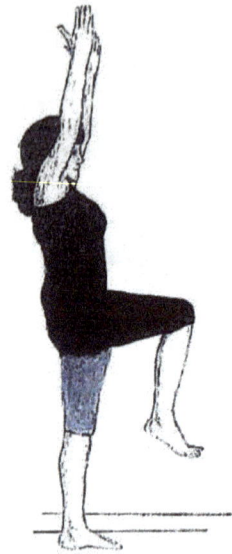

**32**. Prepare to move into a supported **Half Moon** pose. Slide your left/inner palm down the wall as far as you want to go. At the same time, rotate the head and shoulders against the wall. Lift the right/outer leg as high as you can and stretch the upper hand towards the ceiling and look up at it. The upper foot and hand rest on the wall.

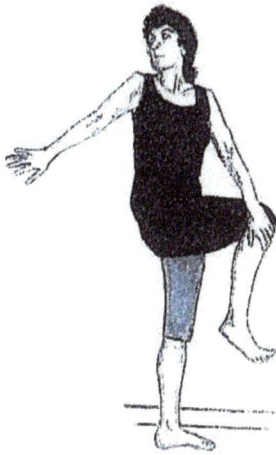

**28**. Place your left/inner hand on the outside of the right/outer knee. Pull the knee towards the wall and twist round in the opposite direction. Slide the palm of the hand along the wall in a supported **Standing Twist**. The head and left/inner shoulder touch the wall. Some people can get both shoulders on the wall.

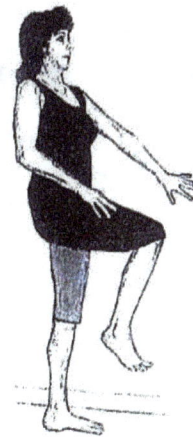

**29**. Move out of the twist and place your right/outer hand on the top of your thigh, in preparation for a supported **Lord of the Dance** pose.

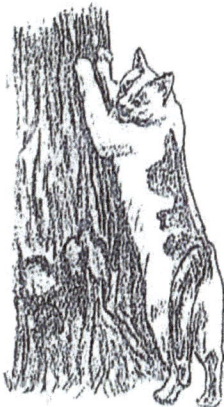

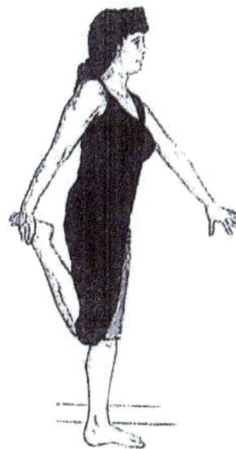

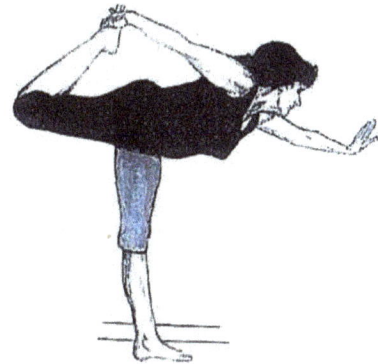

**30**. Slide your hand along the outside of the leg, over the knee and foreleg until you are holding your toes, (some people may prefer to go straight to the toes). Push away with the left/inner palm with the fingers pointing upwards. Look up and lift the foot as high as you can.

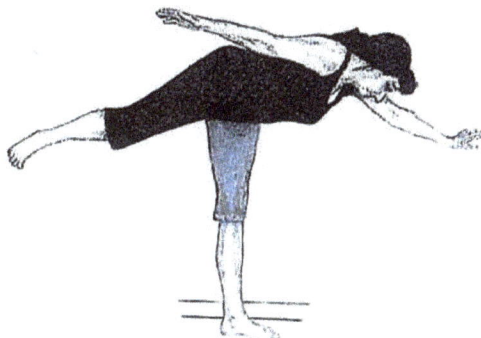

**31**. Take your hand off the foot and straighten the right/outer arm and leg behind. Tilt the front hand towards the floor, look down and push the inner fingers away from the outer toes in a **Diagonal Stretch**. Increase the stretch on the **exhalations** until you feel you have reached your maximum stretch.

# Some ideas for a Restorative Yoga class

My pupils are always pleased to do a **Restorative** class. For newcomers to yoga, this is a class where you use comfortable props to help you get into really restful postures. You stay in the postures for between three and six minutes. It is not necessary to keep absolutely still. I sometimes suggest making slow, meditative movements while improvising in the postures. It does not detract from the relaxation.

I made lots of different shaped bolsters out of pillows and duvets many years ago and they are still fully functional. I give each pupil a clean pillow case at the beginning of class to put around the bolster for hygienic reasons.

I feel it is the energy of the group experience that increases the degree of relaxation achieved in the class. A solo practice does not get the same results. I try not to talk too much and the selection of background music is important. Most melodic music seems too intrusive. Music with different textures seems most relaxing. Most of my pupils like the CD, **Free your Mind** by **Zen Dub**. Also, the music of **Narek Mirzaei** is very impressive and appropriate. Go to www.musicofwisdom.com to hear **Peaceful Breeze** and other examples.

**Tasha**, from **Tranquillity in the City,** taught this restorative version of the **Sphinx** pose at one of her Glastonbury retreats.

Lie on your front and place a bolster under the abdomen to raise it. The feet can be together, with the heels touching, or apart. Place a block, preferably a soft one, so that your forehead is resting on it, as illustrated. It can be tilted so that the top is at a comfortable angle. Rest your forearms on the floor, coming into a supported **Sphinx** pose. When you are ready, slow down your breathing and sink into a dreamy, peaceful state for at least three minutes.

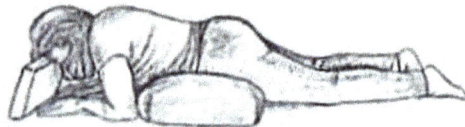

**I improvised** these slow-moving ideas for when the **hips are high up on bolsters**[1]. Start by sitting at the front of the bolster and then slowly lower your back to the floor. If the hips are not high enough, pull the bolster towards you a little. Lift the legs towards the ceiling. Widen the legs out to the side and then take **one minute** to very slowly **move them back together**. This can be part of your time spent in this restorative pose.

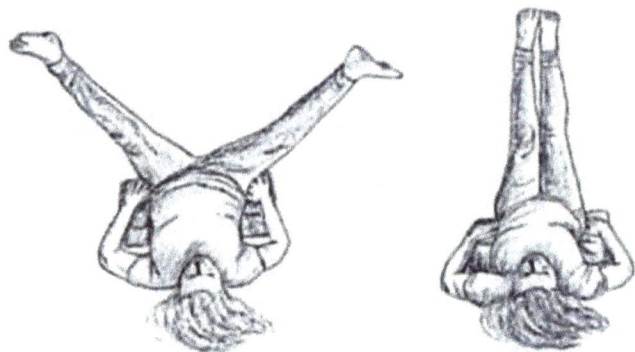

You can also move slowly into a **Supported Half Bridge**. Bring both knees back towards your head and then lower one leg very slowly until first the toes and then the heels, sink into the floor. Take one minute to make the movement, as above. It is interesting to feel the heaviness of the legs in this practice. Bring the leg back and then *change sides and repeat.*

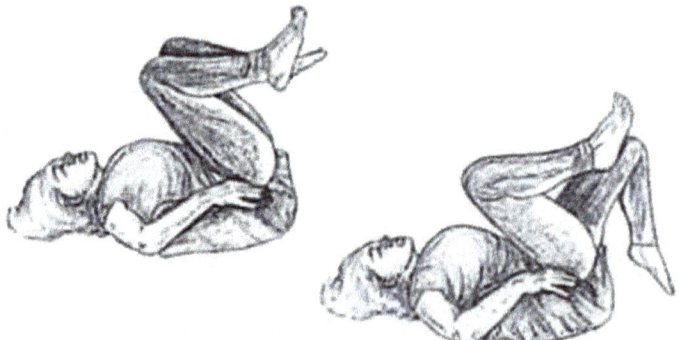

1. Unfortunately, I have mislaid the very good Restorative Yoga DVD I learnt this from many years ago and can't remember who it was by, but it called this restorative pose the **Emperor's Garden** or the **Bamboo Garden.**

*Human beings are part of a whole, called by us 'the universe', a part limited by time and space. One experiences oneself, one's thoughts and feelings as something separate from the rest, which is a kind of optical delusion of consciousness. This delusion is a kind of prison for us, restricting us to our personal desire and the affections of a few persons nearest to us. Our task must be to free ourselves from this prison by widening our circle of compassion to all living creatures and the whole of nature in its beauty. Striving for such an achievement is in itself a part of the liberation and foundation of our inner security.*
**Albert Einstein.**

*The essence of Vedanta is that there is but one Being and that every soul is that being in full, not a part of that being.*

*This grand preaching, the oneness of things, making us one with everything that exists, is the great lesson to learn.*

*Happiness belongs to those who know this oneness, who know they are one with the Universe.* **Swami Vivekananda.**

*In the whole world there is no study so beneficial and so elevating as that of Vedanta.*
**Arthur Schopenhauer**, as quoted at the Vedanta Institute. Comments made after reading the first translations of the ancient Indian scriptures which started to circulate after 1801.

# Introduction to Blocks and Straps Sequence

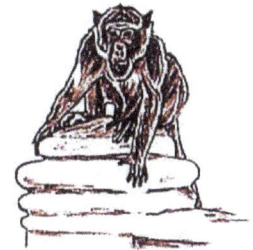

## This is divided into two sections:
## 1. Sequence with Blocks and 2. Sequence with Straps.
### The Sources

I have put these two together because they both came from the same source. At the British Wheel of Yoga Congress, 2019, Zoe Knott taught the postures using blocks and the first five postures with straps in the second section. This inspired me to expand the ideas into these sequences.

In **Sequence with Straps, Variations A** and **B** are my ideas. Please read the information about the importance of standing on one leg in the box below.

I came across similar postures to those in **Variation C** in books by two teachers who had studied with B.K.S Iyengar. They are **A Chair for Yoga** by **Eyal Shifroni** and **How to Use Yoga** by **Mira Mehta**[1].

The **Lord of the Dance, Boat** and **Pretzel** poses with straps, all come from general yogic repertoire.

### Additional Notes

I must confess that I have never had to buy yoga straps because my father left so many ties in his wardrobe. My pupils have found them adequate but they are not long enough for very tall people. Obviously, you can do more things with a purpose-made yoga strap.

The sequence with blocks is for every age group. I have used a child to model it because he looks so cute in the postures. He is my youngest pupil. I have been teaching him since he was three and a half years old.

**Bone density and strength** are improved by stress on the bone. When astronauts go up in space, they return with reduced bone density. This is because they did not experience the pull of gravity high above planet Earth.

**Standing on one leg**, in a constructive way, improves balance and decreases the risk of spontaneous falls. It also strengthens the bone and minimises the chance of a fracture if a person falls.

1. **A Chair for Yoga** by **Eyal Shifroni**, 2014, published by CreateSpace Independent Publishing Platform. It can be purchased by visiting www.achairyoga.com **How to use Yoga** by Mira Mehta, 1994. by Anness Publishing, Select Editions.

# 1. Sequence with Blocks

**Hold all postures for a few breaths or longer if you choose to.**

**1.** Stand with the feet a hip-width apart and place your hands on your hips.

**2.** Lift the chest and lean backwards.

**3.** Slowly return to **1**. Lower from the tops of the thighs until the trunk is parallel to the floor.

**4.** Bend the knees, sinking the hips backwards. Bring the chest towards the thighs and feel the stretch on the lower spine.

**5.** Move the feet together as you catch hold of your block. Position it on its side in front of you, far enough away for your arms to be straight with the fingertips on top of the block.

**6.** Sink down into the squat and stretch the right hand away, hovering over or beyond the block.

**7.** Move your right hand to the outside of the left lower leg. Push up on your left fingertips and twist round to the left, looking up under the armpit.

**8.** When you are ready, straighten the legs and continue to twist round to the left.

**9.** Rotate forwards with both hands on the block again. Return to your squatting posture, as in **4**. ***Change side and repeat.***

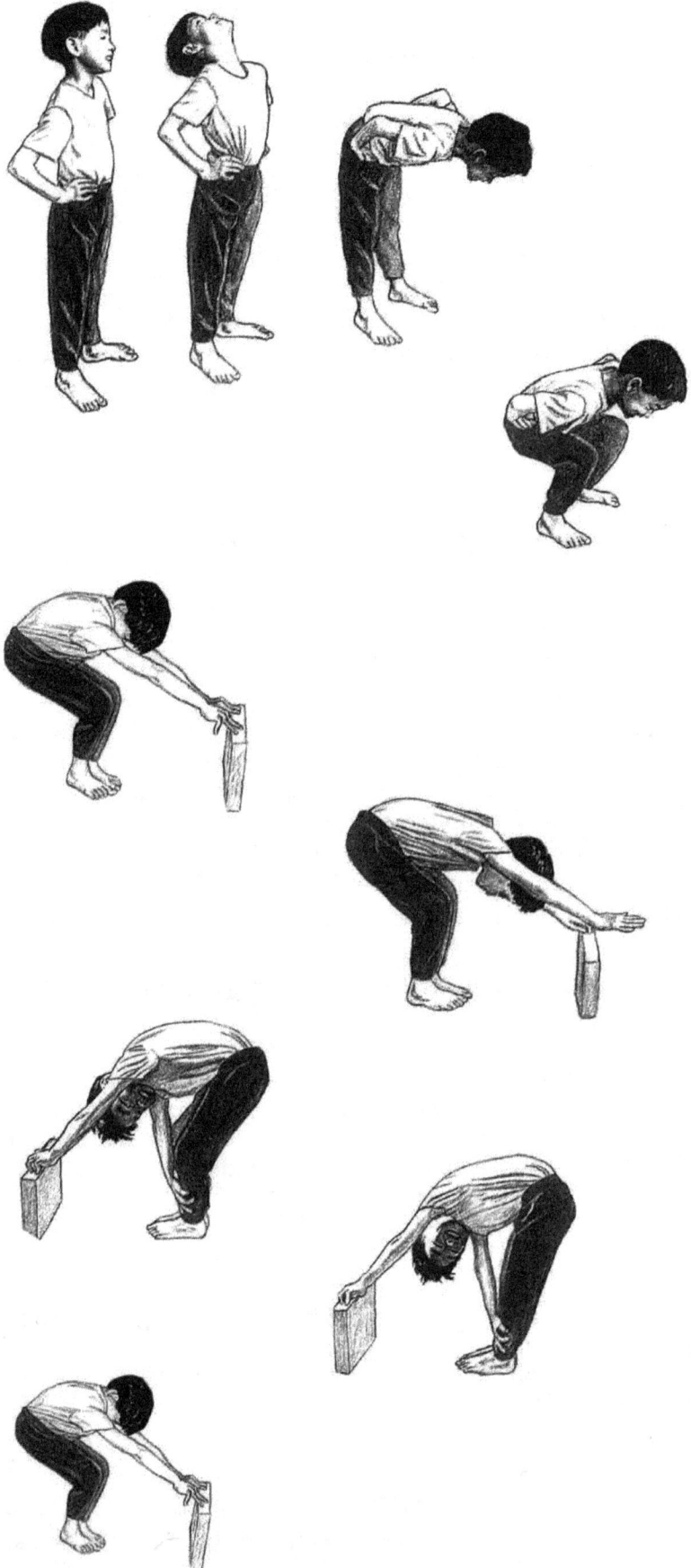

**10**. When you have worked through to **9** again on the other side, move the block to one side and place the fingertips on the floor with the knees bent. After a few breaths, straighten the legs. Move the finger tips a little closer if you need to. When the time is right, lower your palms to the floor.

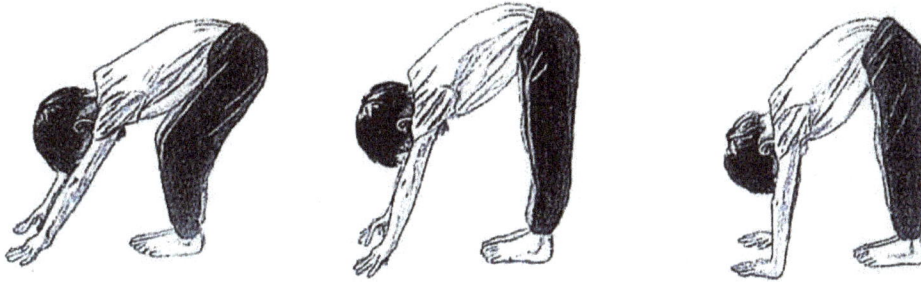

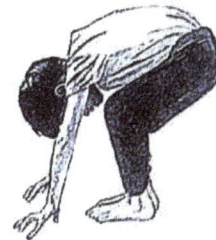

*Repeat this once more* with the fingers closer to the feet.
Remember: *Fingertips to the floor,* knees bent
*Fingertips to the floor,* knees straight
*Palms to the floor*

**11**. Lower into the squat again and place the hands low down on the backs of the legs. Try to relax. Feel the body yielding to the posture and the heaviness of the head.

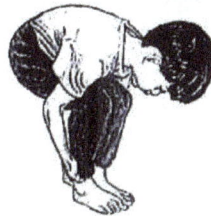

**To return to 1** we are going to repeat the **first three postures in reverse**. You may choose to keep the feet together.

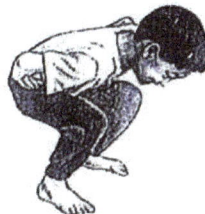

Place your hands on your hips.

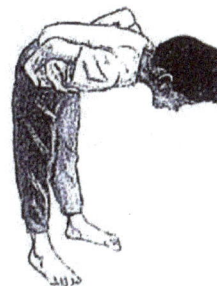

Straighten the legs and return to **3**.

Slowly raise the head and lift the chest, retuning to **2**.

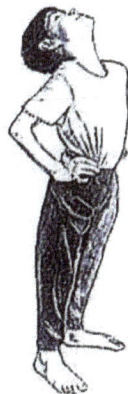

Return to **1** and bring your hands into **Prayer**.

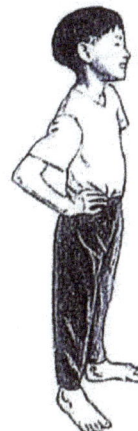

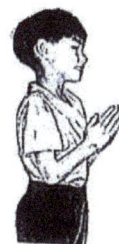

**Now repeat from 1 to 10 but, this time, with your feet wide apart.**
Some experimentation may be necessary to gauge the most beneficial width. Make them as wide apart as you comfortably can.
The instructions will be the same until **6**, when you can add a twist in the opposite direction. In **7**, the hand will need to be higher up the lower leg.

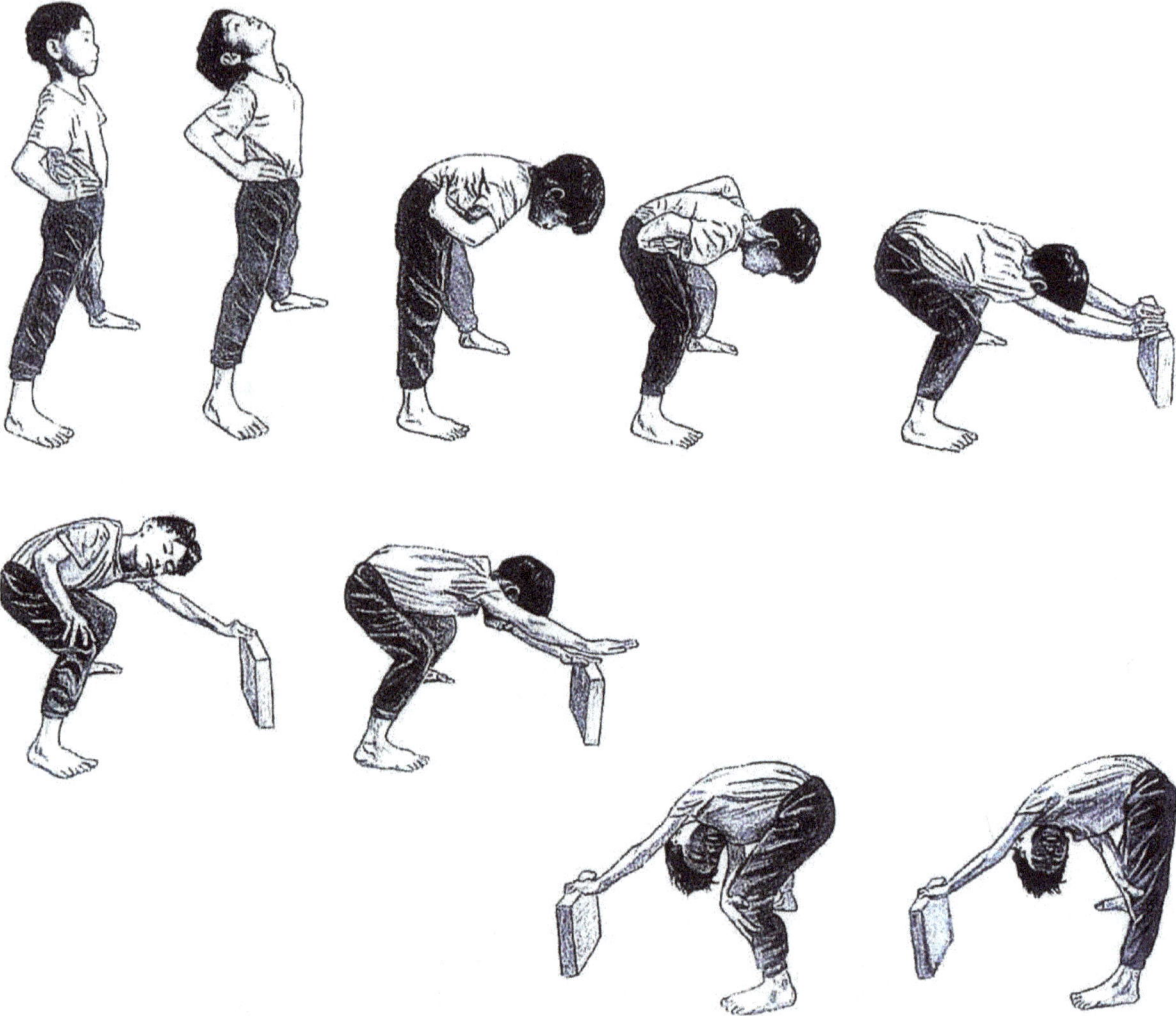

*Change sides and repeat from 4 to 9.*

**When you get to 10**, remove the block as before and repeat the procedure with the hands stretched out in front.

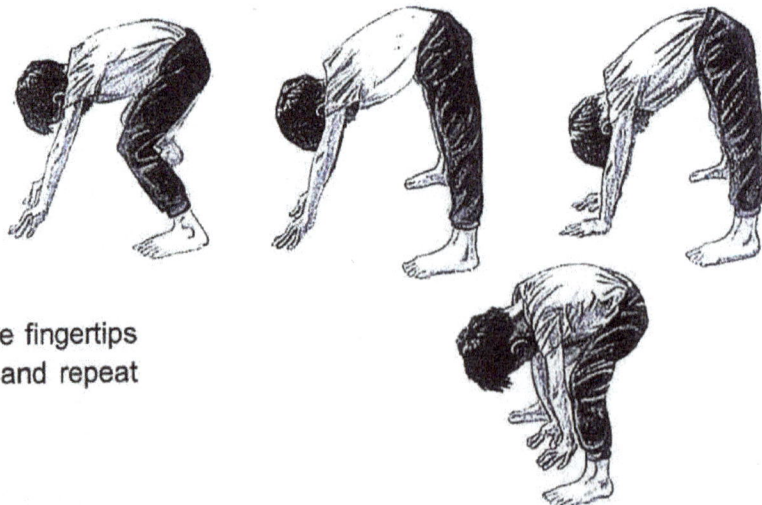

**The second time**, bring the fingertips back in line with the feet and repeat as above.

Repeat it a **third time** with the hands through the legs, rotated and pointing backwards.

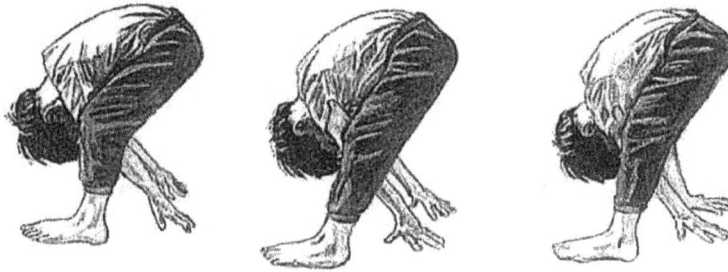

**To conclude**, return to **11**. The elbows can be on the outside of the knees.

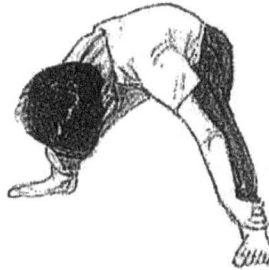

Repeat the introduction in reverse with the feet wide apart.

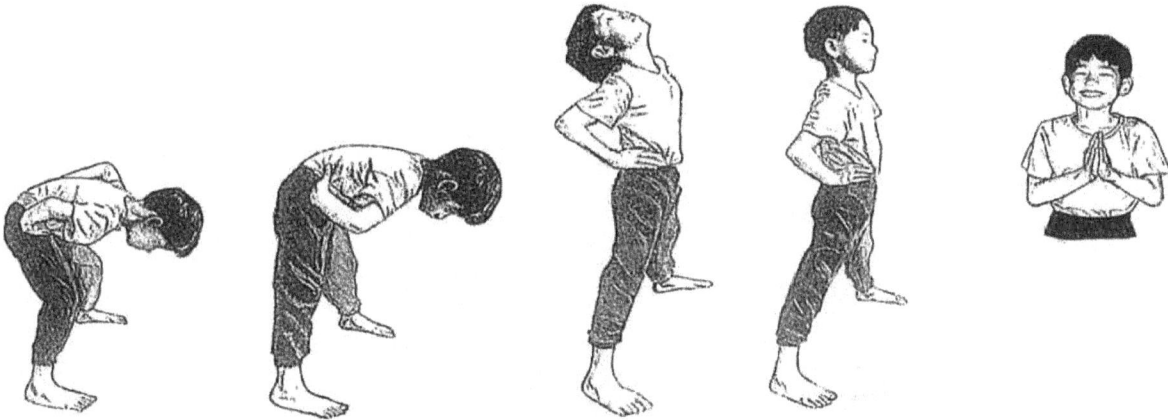

**Variations**. Some body types will need to improvise with different props. For example, if you have very long legs you can use a chair instead of a block and increase the number of blocks used if necessary, as illustrated below.

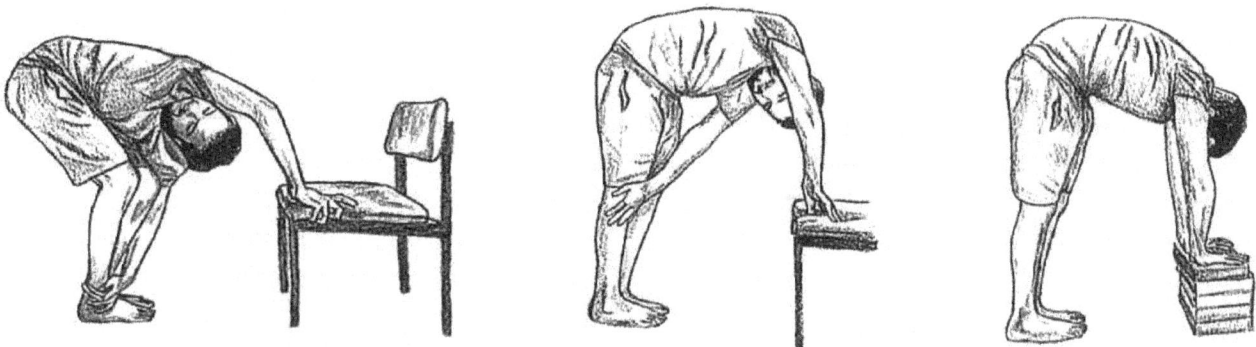

## 2. Yoga with Straps

1. Stand with the feet hip-width apart. Catch hold of your strap and hold it above your head with the hands shoulder-width apart.

2. **INHALE** as you stretch the hands upwards. **EXHALE** as you lean over to the right. Hold for a few breaths, slowly increasing the stretch.
*Change sides and repeat.*

3. Come back to centre with your hands above your head. **INHALE** as you lift the chest, without lifting the shoulders, pushing up from the point between the shoulder blades. The head will automatically move backwards but the neck will still be in line with the spine.
Hold for a few breaths.

4. Widen the distance between the hands by about 6 - 9 inches (16 - 23 cm.). We are going to stretch up the right side and open up the right armpit. One of my pupils called this **Armpit Liberation** and the name stuck.
Bring your left hand out to the side and back and pull the right arm back.
Hold for a few breaths. *Change sides and repeat.*

5. Bring the strap behind your back. Catch hold of it with the hands shoulder-width apart. **INHALE** as you lift the hands. Hold for a few breaths, slowly lifting the hands higher.

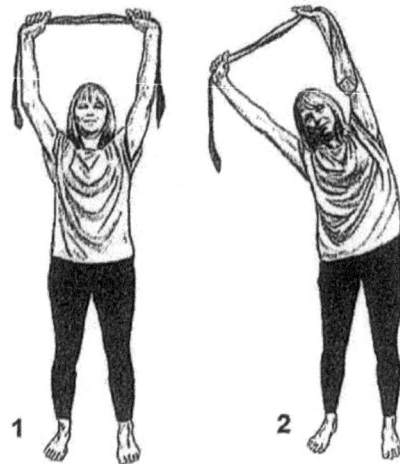

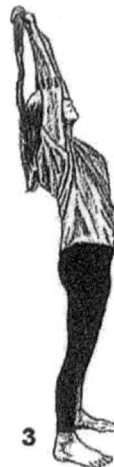

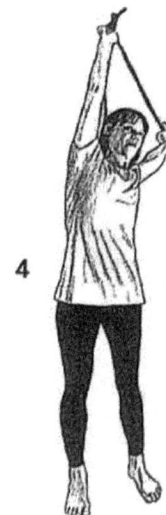

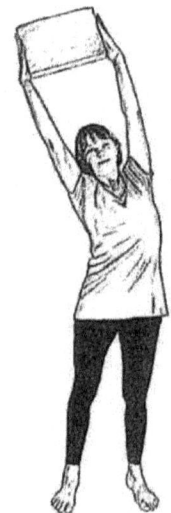

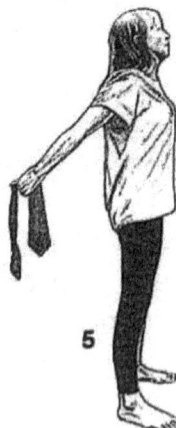

## Variations

**You can use a block** instead of a strap for these two pages.

**A. Repeat the above sequence with a chair.**
As the shape of chairs varies, you will have to adjust your foot position to the chair you are using. Ideally, push the chair against a wall and place your heel on the chair and your toes on the back of the chair, or on the wall if there is a gap. The foot of the supporting leg faces the chair. Straighten the leg on the chair. When you feel secure and comfortable, catch hold of the strap and repeat the sequence from **2** to **5**.
**Caution.** If you have back or leg problems, proceed with caution. Stop if there is any discomfort. In a beginners or mixed ability class, you may choose to change legs before you get to **5**.

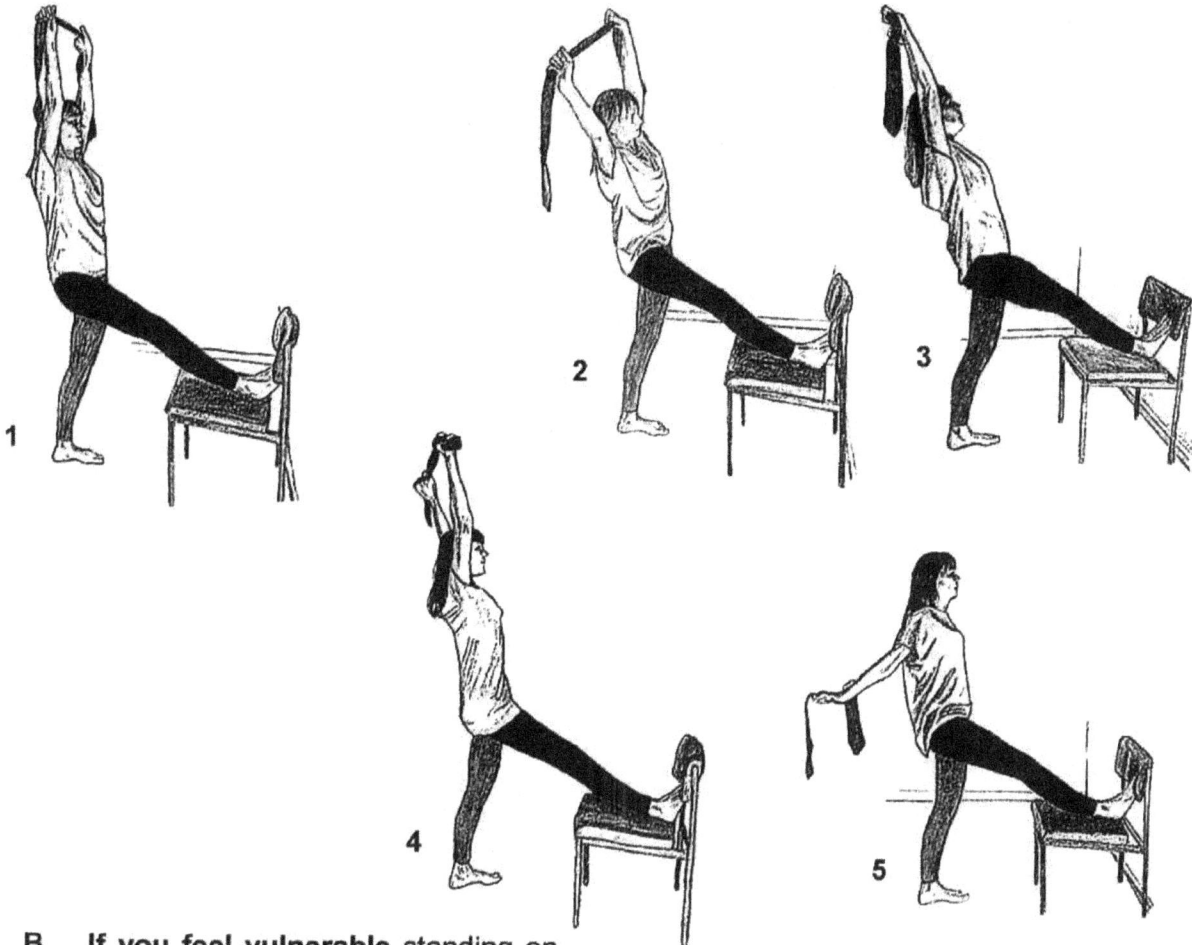

B.  **If you feel vulnerable** standing on one leg, you can stand with your back against a wall.  Place the chair on a yoga mat in front of you so it can't slip.

In **3**, you can lean forwards a little. In **4**, the arm that is behind will need to go further out to the side, and in **5**, you will need to lean forwards so that you can lift your hands behind your back.

Start with the heel of the supporting leg about 6 inches away from the wall.  You can keep your hips on the wall throughout the sequence.

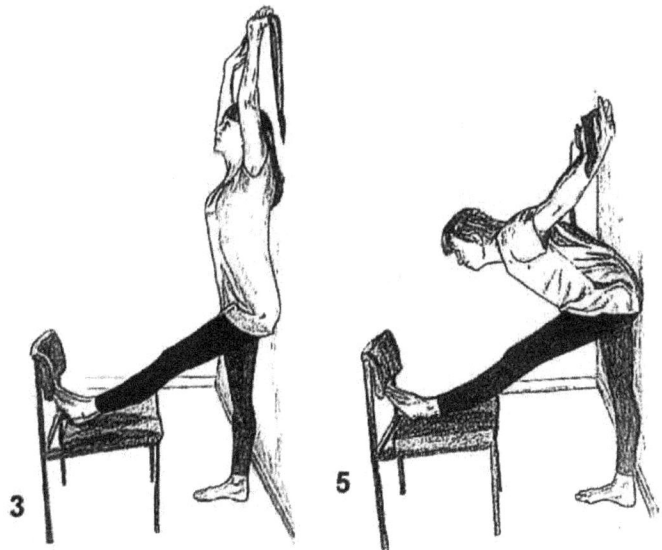

**Before you change sides**, rest in this **restorative pose** for as long as you want to.  If you need to rest your legs, you could rest in **Child's Pose**.

Stand with the feet wide apart and place your forearms on the chair.  Rest your forehead on your hands, the chair, cushion or bolster.  It is very relaxing to rest the forehead on something soft and comfortable.  **If you have high blood pressure**, turn the chair around and rest your forearms on the back of the chair and repeat the procedure.  *Change sides and repeat this variation.*

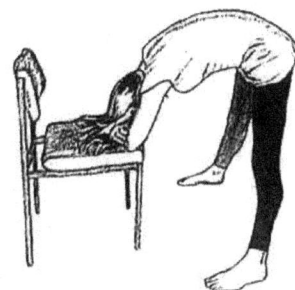

**C.** As in the previous variation, you can change legs when you need to. **Hold each posture between 25 and 60 seconds**.

We are going to lift one leg up at roughly a 90 degree angle to the supporting leg. If you are lucky enough to have a secure ledge, you can use that. An appropriate piece of furniture, e.g., a table or a stool with a block on top, pushed against a wall will also suffice. If you are using the top of the back of a chair, push it against a wall. You may need to place a blanket or something similar under your foot for comfort and to create a little distance from the wall.

Before you lift your leg up, make a loop at the end of your strap large enough for one foot to pass through it. If you are using a tie, make a knot in it. Face the chair and place the loop around your right foot. Lift the foot up onto your support and position the loop around the ball of your foot. **When you are secure and comfortable** you may begin.

**1.** Hold the strap with both hands and stretch the top of your head up towards the ceiling.

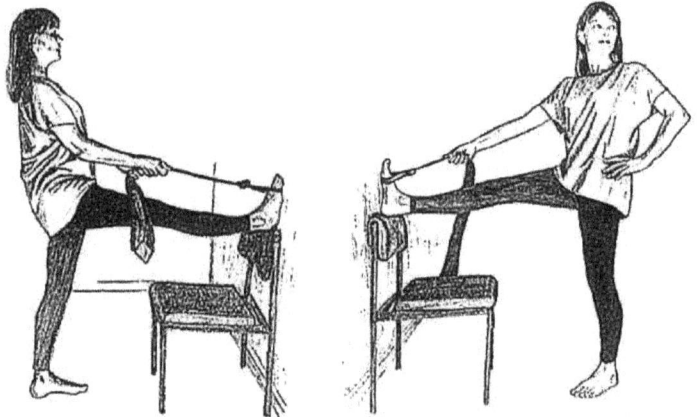

**2.** Turn your left foot to a 45 degree angle. Catch hold of the strap with your right hand, place your left hand on your hip and twist round to the left.

**3.** Stay facing sideways. **INHALE** the left arm up and **EXHALE** it towards the wall. Rotate your left shoulder back and look up to the left. You can rest your right elbow on the leg.
You may choose to shorten the strap a little by moving your hand up the strap towards the loop.

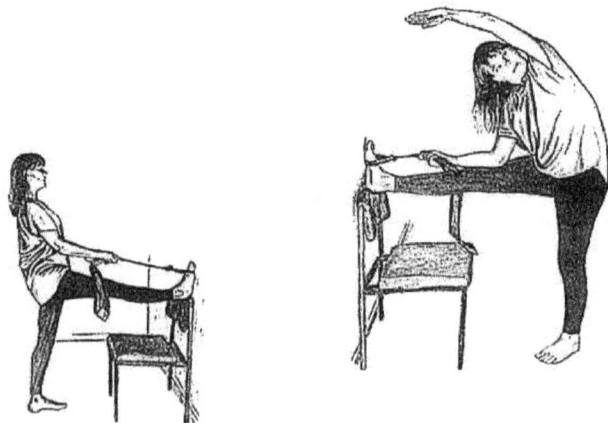

**4.** Return to **1**.

**5.** Catch hold of your strap with your left hand and twist round to the right. Place the right hand on your hip. Stretch the top of your head up towards the ceiling, as before.

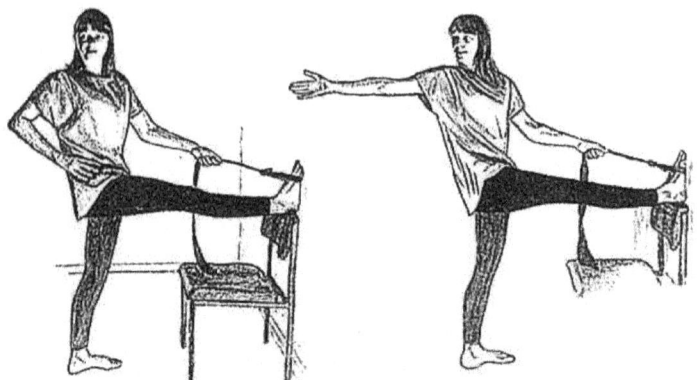

**6.** Stretch your right hand out to the side and twist round a bit more.

**If you have not changed legs**, return to the **Restorative posture** on the previous page before changing sides.

# Lord of the Dance Posture with Straps

Make a loop in your strap big enough for your foot to pass through. One tie will not be long enough if you're a tall person. You will have to use a yoga strap. If you haven't got one, you can improvise with two ties tied together or something similar.

We start against a wall as most people find the free-standing version too challenging.

**I have not suggested how long you hold the postures for.** That will depend on individual levels of fitness and general constitution. **Come out of the posture carefully** if there is any discomfort.

**1**. Start with your right shoulder close to the wall. Lift the right foot in front and place the loop around the ball of the foot. Carefully move the foot behind[1] you and bring the strap over your right shoulder. If the strap moves too far down the foot, adjust it before you proceed.

First hold the strap with both hands. Lean forwards a little and pull on the strap until you have raised your right foot to a reasonable height.

When you are ready, hold the strap with your right hand and stretch the left hand forward.

**2**. Hold the strap with both hands again and bring it over the head to the left shoulder. Repeat the procedure, first holding with both hands and then holding with the left hand and stretching along the wall with your right hand.

**3**. Hold the strap with both hands again and bring it up over your head. Hold for as long as you choose, slowly pulling the foot higher. You can vary this by holding the strap with one hand and stretching the other one forward if you choose to.

**Rest in an appropriate posture** before changing side if you need to or:
*Change side and repeat*.

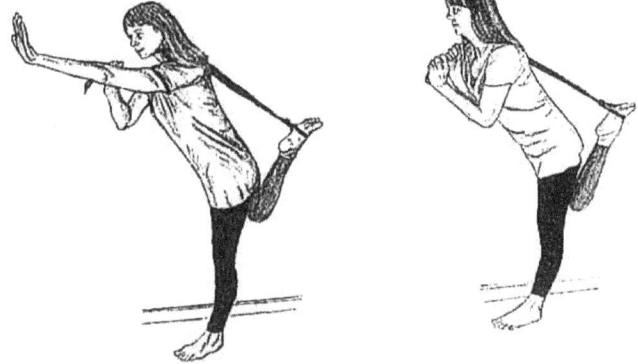

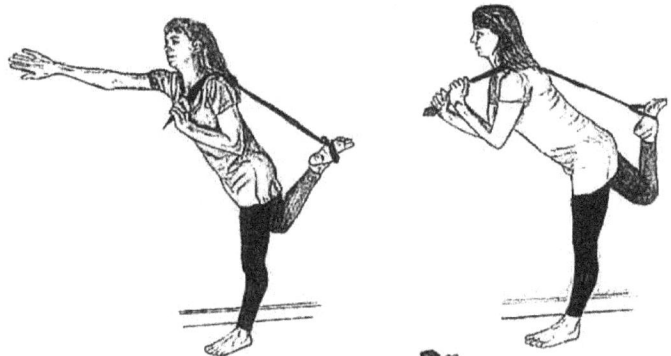

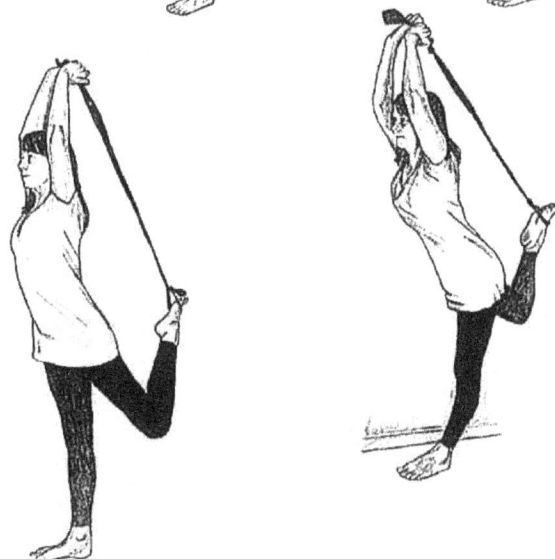

**4. Only try it free standing** if you feel you can rise to the challenge.

1. When I was experimenting with this variation my foot landed heavily on the floor and I stubbed my toes. The discomfort lasted for a few weeks. If somebody has bad coordination, it may be necessary to pair up with a helper and take it in turns to practise and assist.

## Boat Pose with Straps

You do not need a loop in the end of your strap for this practice. If you are using a tie, place the wid
part of the tie around your feet.

**1.** Sit with your feet together and the knees bent. Place your strap around the balls of your feet and hold it with both hands. Slowly lift the feet off the ground, keeping the knees bent and then straighten the legs. **Hold for a few breaths**.

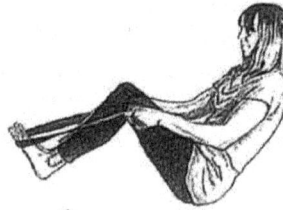

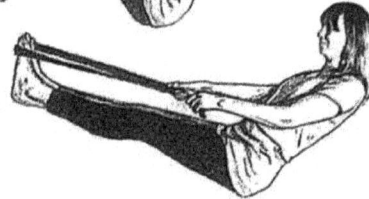

**2.** Hold the strap in your right hand and stretch the left hand round and back, twisting to the left. Increase the twist by moving the legs to the right. You can lower the left hand to the floor. **Hold for a few breaths and return to 1**.

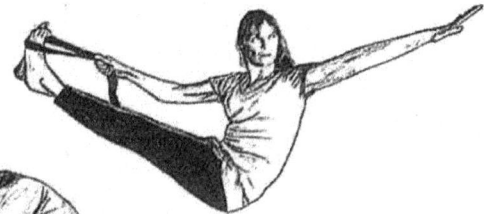

**Rest if you need to** by folding forwards with the elbows between the knees and catching hold of the feet in the **Resting Butterfly**. *Change sides and repeat.*

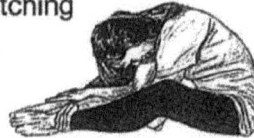

## Pretzel Pose[1] with Straps

I came across this pose practised in different ways with straps on various sites on the internet. For more information about it go to the **Piriformis Stretch Sequence** on page **77**

**1.** Make a loop in your strap. Lie on your back with the knees bent. Place the loop over the ball of your right foot. Lift the left ankle over the right knee, keeping the strap above the leg. Lift the right foot off the floor and pull the strap towards the head with both hands. To increase the stretch, you can hold the strap in your right hand and push the left knee away with your left hand. You are likely to feel a stretch on the side of your left hip. This is explained on page **75**

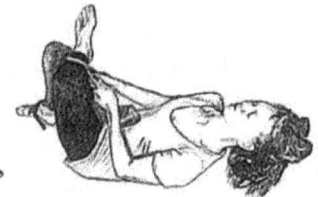

**Hold for a few breaths** and then straighten the right leg. Shorten the strap and continue to pull the leg towards the head.

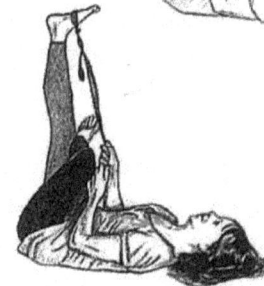

**When the time is right**, lift the head and shoulders. You can lower the right leg after a few breaths and find your maximum stretch in this pose.

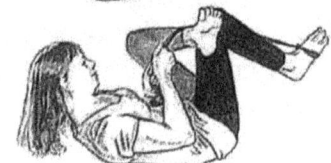

**2.** Remove the loop from the right foot and place it round the ball of your left foot and lift the foot on to the right knee. Lift the right foot off the floor and pull the strap with both hands towards your head. You can push the left knee away with your left hand, as above, if you choose.

**Hold for a few breaths** and then lift the head and shoulders and pull the foot closer to your head again, increasing the stretch on the side of the left hip. Straightening the right leg is not necessary when the strap is on the left foot.

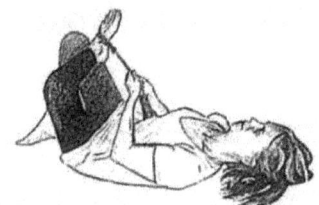

**3.** Remove the loop from your left foot and place the wide part of the tie or strap around the back of your right thigh. Place the left ankle over the right knee again and lift the right foot. Hold the strap with both hands close to the thigh and pull the leg back towards your head. Move the left knee in the opposite direction and feel the same stretch again. **Repeat as in 1**, straightening the right leg and then lifting the head and shoulders.
*Change sides and repeat*

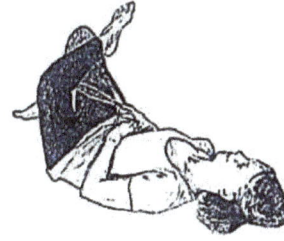

1. I have always known this pose as **Pretzel Pose** but I know it has other names. Some other postures are also called **Pretzel Pose** so the name is rather ambiguous.

## More about Vedanta

**According to Vedanta**, knowledge is of two kinds: (1) The perfect experience of consciousness[1]; (2) The knowledge of objects, or the ordinary imperfect experience of the world owing to the association with the mind[2].

Shankara's[3] explanation of the relation between the absolute and the finite world[4] is expressed in the story of the snake and the rope.

*In the darkness, one mistakes the rope for a snake. When a light is brought, the illusion of the snake created by the lack of illumination is removed, and once again the rope appears in its true reality. So, also, the world is only a superimposition on Brahman[5], the absolute. Owing to ignorance, man thinks of the existence of the finite world like a snake in darkness. When the knowledge of oneness dawns, the world disappears, and once again only the absolute exists.*

From *The Complete Illustrated Book of Yoga* by Swami Vishnu Devananda, 1960, Three Rivers Press

### LOOK AND FIND ME

Look at a cup of tea,
There you will find me.

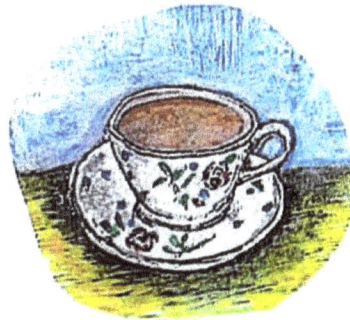

Look at the sun,
There I am.

Look at a flower,
There you will find me.

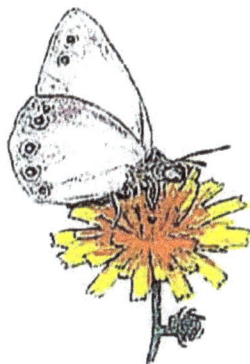

Look at a river,
There I am.

Look at the fire,
There you will find me.

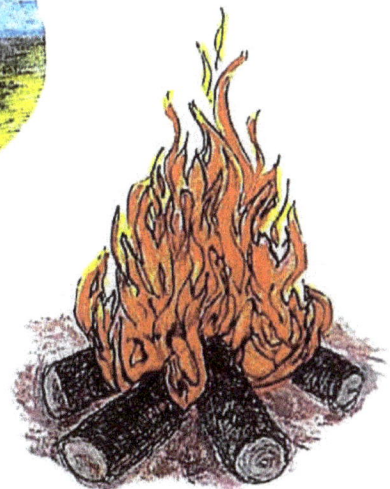

Swami Sivananda, 1887-1963.

1. *Gyana swaroopa* in Sanskrit. **2.** *Gyana vritti* in Sanskrit. **3.** See page 48. **4.** *Vivarta Vada* in *Sanskrit*.
5. *Brahman* is the Hindu equivalent of God. I prefer to use 'Divine energy' instead of the word God.

# The Necessity for Caution when Putting the Head Back

*The neck is composed of seven vertebrae stacked upon each other to provide support and movement to the head. This arrangement provides flexibility and a lot of movement to permit correct positioning to the sense organs in space (eyes, ears, nose and mouth). The neck also carries major vital structures to and from the brain to the body. Important arteries and veins, air pipes and nerves commanding movements of the body and its vital functions, are carried in the neck with hardly any major structural protection surrounding them. This is because a hard and bony cage would mean loss of range of movement that is so necessary in this anatomical region.*

*It is important therefore to understand the relationship between maintaining a healthy level of movement and flexibility of function of the neck, whilst being very careful and mindful of these vital structures passing between joints and underneath muscles.*

*Accidents, falls and genetic abnormalities cause the neck to become even more vulnerable to instability and possible compression of nerves and vessels. When exercising it is therefore paramount to listen to one's body. Signs like dizziness, light-headedness, visual changes, tingling or numbness in the limbs, sharp pain or difficulty swallowing are major red flags and indicate that you need to swiftly stop any exercise and seek medical help.*

*If you have suffered with previous neck issues, car accidents, vertigo when turning the head, or are taking medications, it is advisable to ask your GP for advice before starting any exercises, especially when they involve arching and/or deeply rotating the head backwards. This particular combination of movements – backward arching and rotation of the neck – put strain and compression on one of the vessels taking blood to the brain, the vertebral artery. This artery is very easily injured with very unpleasant consequences, including strokes.*

*It is therefore very important to keep in mind this gentle structure when exercising and doing this particular set of movements and, if in doubt in regard to the health of your neck, avoid them altogether until you have consulted a health professional.*

*A great way to get the benefits of this practice without physically engaging in the techniques is to mentally visualise and perform each movement in your mind's eye. Imagine and* **see** *your body going through the full sequence. Spend the same amount of time* **observing** *your body freely doing each of the listed movements and* **hold** *the pose for the suggested times. This will give you very similar benefits without any of the possible complications.*

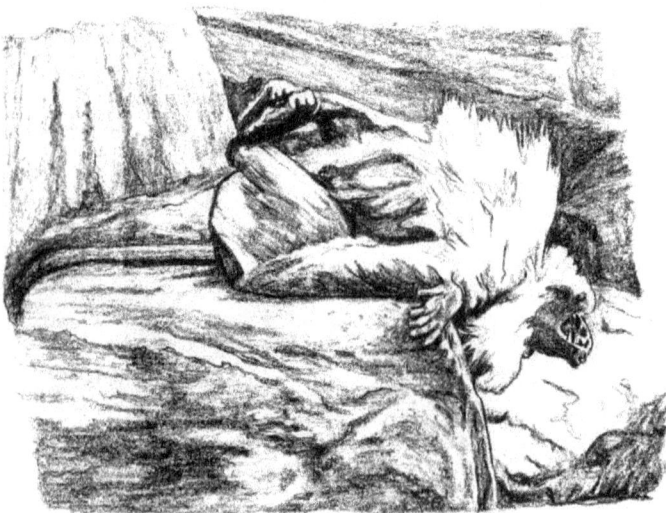

*However, it is important not to become too fearful to use the body in healthy and expressive ways. Therefore, before limiting your practice with unnecessary worries, do consult a GP and ask their permission to perform the postures in the* **Heart Opening Sequence** *and just be gentle and mindful with your movements.*
*Good luck with your practice!*

Elisa Burato M.Ost.
kuulondon.co.uk

A baboon hanging with its head back over a ledge.

# Introduction to the Piriformis Stretch Sequence

I don't usually get involved with individual muscles when I teach yoga but the **piriformis**[1] is an exception. When it shortens for various reasons, or is too tight, this can put pressure on the **sciatic nerve**. **Piriformis Syndrome** occurs when the piriformis irritates the sciatic nerve.

A tight piriformis can also cause discomfort lower down in the legs. After we did this sequence in one class, a lady who had some sciatic pain said it had disappeared, and another one said her bad knee was less troublesome.

---

The sciatic nerve is the longest in the body and is as thick as your index finger. It usually runs under the piriformis muscle. In 17% of people it passes through the piriformis muscle. These people are predisposed to developing sciatica. This is not the only cause of sciatica but it can be a contributory factor.

Sciatica can be described as pain, tingling or numbness deep in the buttocks and along the sciatic nerve.

---

Most people will feel an easily identifiable stretch on the hip when the piriformis muscle is being stretched. I have started off the sequence with the stretches using chairs because these are the best ones for locating this stretch.

A few people won't feel the stretch. This is most probably because their piriformis muscle is already stretched. When I did this sequence in my **U3A**[2] class, a very flexible pupil of 78 years told me she couldn't feel the stretches that the rest of the class were feeling abundantly. After the class, she told me that when she watches television, she sits on her sofa with one foot behind her head. She doesn't put two feet up in case she gets stuck. She says her grandchildren think she is very weird. Unfortunately, she didn't want me to take a photo of her sitting like that for this book!

## Sources of the Postures

I had come across **1** and **2** a few times in books and workshops, but not **3**. They are all explained well in **Kristin McGee's** book **Chair Yoga**. Variations of **4** can be found on numerous videos on the internet. **Pretzel Pose** (often called other names) is from general yogic repertoire. **6** comes from a video by **Ron Miller PT**, called **Sciatica Exercise for Piriformis Syndrome**. **7** comes from a video by **Dr James Vegher** called **One movement for Instant Sciatica Pain Relief**. **8** is described by several people on the internet. **9** is from general yogic repertoire.

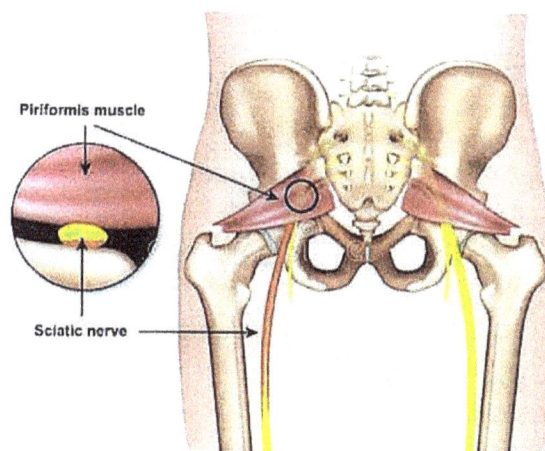

Royalty Free Vector Image

1. The name of the muscle comes from the Latin *Piriformis*, meaning *pear*-shaped.
2. U3A is the **University of the Third Age**. It is for people over 60 years old.

# Piriformis Stretch Sequence

**1.** Stand a short distance behind a chair with the feet together. Place your hands on the back of the chair. Bend the knees and place the left ankle over the right knee.

Sink down into a squat. You are likely to feel a stretch on the outside of your left hip. If you don't feel it, move the left knee towards the floor and squat down a bit further. You can push it down gently with your left hand. **This is where you will feel your Piriformis stretches.**
*Change sides and repeat.*
**Variation**

Hold the back of the chair with your right hand and turn to the side. Repeat the procedure, as illustrated.

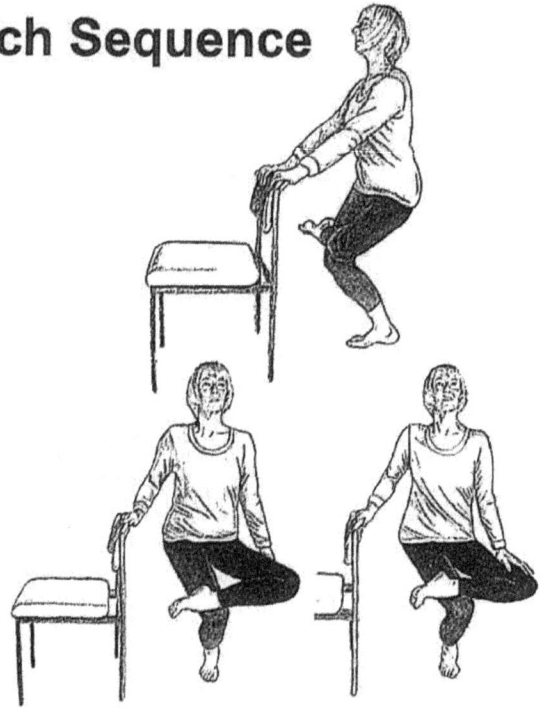

**2.** Sit as far to the front of the chair as you comfortably can, with the feet together. Place the left ankle on the right knee again. You can keep your right hand on the ankle and push the left knee towards the floor with your left hand if necessary.

Keeping the spine in a neutral position, slowly lean forwards until you feel the stretch on the left hip. To increase the stretch, push the knee down with your left hand and lean further forwards.
**Variation**

You can place both forearms on the left leg while you are lowering down and then let the arms dangle as you hold the posture.
*Change sides and repeat.*

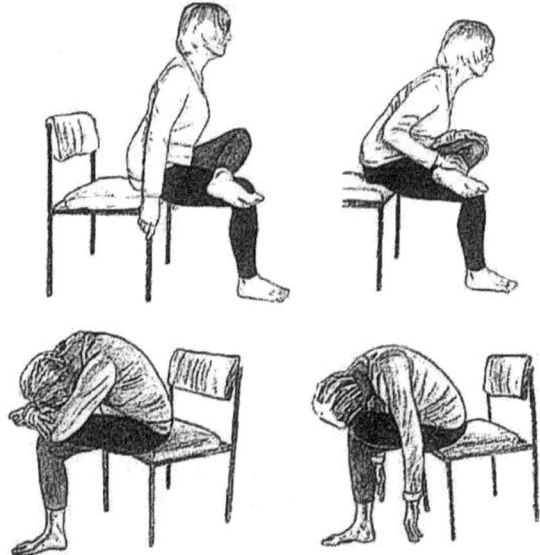

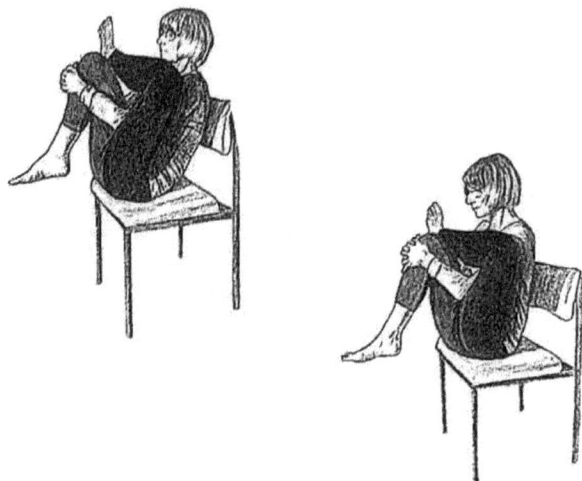

**3.** Your ease in establishing the next posture will depend on your arm-to-body ratio. If you have short arms, it will help if you lean your shoulders on the back of the chair and slide as far to the front of the chair as you safely can.

Place your left ankle on the right knee and slowly lift the legs while moving the shoulders towards the back of the chair. Keep the spine in a neutral position. Slide your left arm between the legs and along the inside of the right thigh and join the hands together on the front of the right knee. If you can't reach the front of the knee, go for the back of the right thigh. Pull the legs back as far as you can.

If you have long arms, you may be able to join your hands together on the front of your knee before you lift the legs up. You may also be able to hold the stretch without leaning backwards.
*Change sides and repeat.*

## 4. Knee to Opposite Shoulder Stretch

This has several variations. We will stay on the chair for the first one. Your arm-to-body ratio will influence how you hold your leg to get the best stretch. Tall, slim people will find the stretch easier to move into. Tummies may get in the way. Hold each variation for as long as you choose.

**A.** Sit up straight on the front of the chair with the feet together. Lift the left knee, hold it with both hands and pull it up and over towards the right shoulder. To increase the stretch, move the right hand further down the leg and pull the foreleg towards the right shoulder.
*Change sides and repeat.*

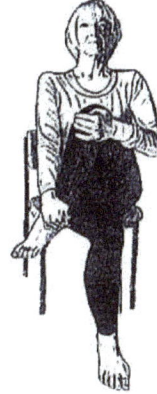

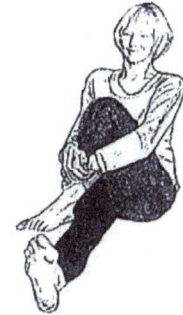

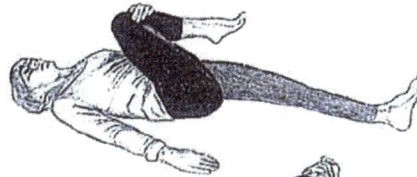

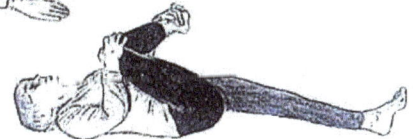

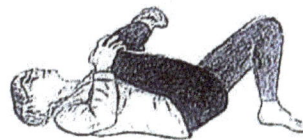

**B.** Sit on your mat with the right leg straight in front. Pick up your left knee and pull it over to your right shoulder, as above. Sit up straight and keep both hips on the floor. Move the right hand down the leg, as above, if necessary.
*Change sides and repeat*

**C.** Lie on your back with both legs straight. Bring your right knee back, catch hold of it and pull it back towards your left shoulder. From this point, you can experiment.
 You can hold it back with one hand or hold with two and pull the foreleg back.
 You can bend the left knee and keep the foot on the floor or lift it a little off the floor and then straighten the leg towards the ceiling.
*Change sides and repeat.*

## 5. Pretzel Pose

Lie on your back again. Bend the left knee and place your right ankle on the left knee. Lift your head, shoulders and left foot. Move your right arm along the inside of your left thigh and interlock the fingers on the front of the left knee. Bring your head towards your knee.
Push the right knee away with your right hand to increase the stretch.
Most people will feel a powerful **Piriformis stretch** in this posture. To practise it with **straps**, turn to page **72**

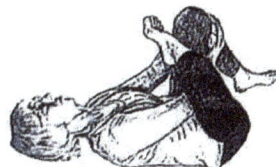

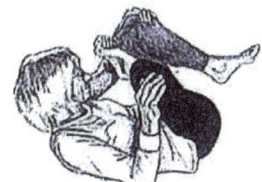

## 6. Four Points Stretch

Come onto all fours with the knees close together and the hands under the shoulders. Keeping the knees in the same place, move the lower legs over to the left. Stretch the left leg back over the right leg, resting the toes on the floor.

**Move your hips over to the right.** This brings your left shoulder towards your right knee. You can bend the elbows, rotate the hands inwards and lower the head to increase the stretch. Hold for at least 20 seconds.

*Change sides and repeat.*

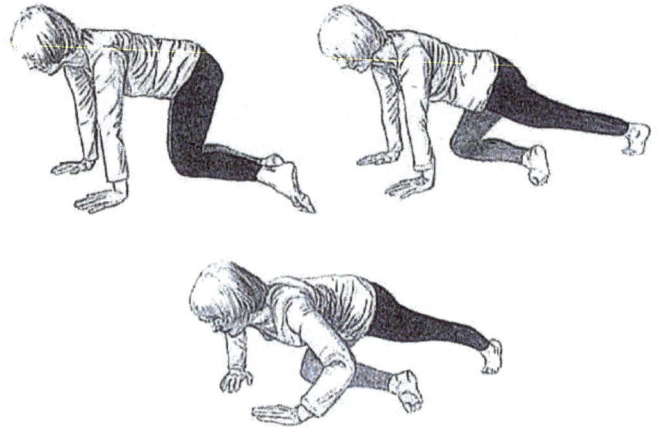

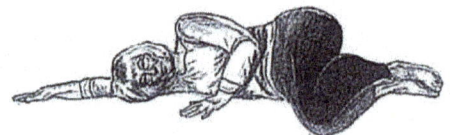

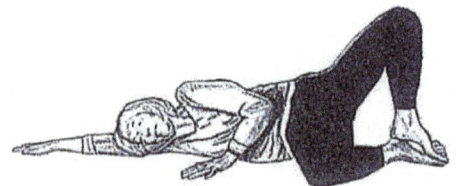

## 7. Hand and Knee Slide

Lie on your right side with your top shoulder directly above your bottom one. Support your head with a block, or something similar. The knees are bent and forwards, roughly at a right angle to the body. The thighs are parallel to the arms which are in front with the hands in **Prayer**.

**Slide your top hand and knee away from you**, ensuring they move the same distance, until you feel a **stretch across the bottom hip**. Hold for a few breaths while you experience the stretch. Repeat a few times and then hold for a little longer.

It is similar to the other stretches in the sequence but you are stretching from a different direction. *Change sides and repeat.*

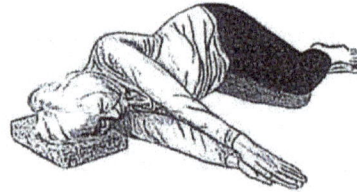

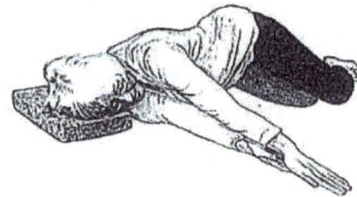

## 8. Clam Pose

We are not *stretching* the muscle in this posture, we are *contracting* it.

Stay on your right side, stretch your right arm along the floor and rest your head on your upper arm. Keep your knees bent and forwards, as above. Rest your left hand or fingertips on the floor in front of your waist.

INHALE as you open the left knee up towards the ceiling. Do not move the hip back. Hold for a few breaths while you experience the **contracted Piriformis muscle**.

EXHALE the knee down and repeat a few times until the feeling becomes familiar.

Some health professionals recommend holding the knee up for **one minute**. Choose the time that feels right for you.

*Change sides and repeat.*

**Variations**

You can rest your head on your hand and place the left hand on the hip, on the area where you feel the compression.

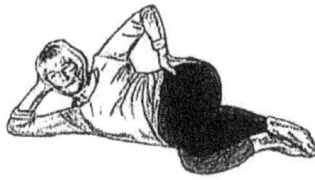

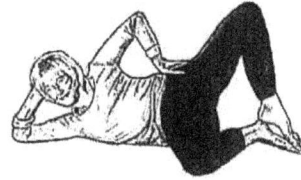

You can lie length ways along a wall with all parts of your back very close to it. This will help you keep your hips in line and encourage you to open your knees a little more.

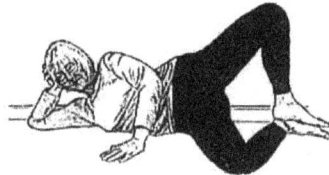

### 9. Sitting sideways against the wall

Sit sideways against a wall with your inner hip and knee touching the wall. Roll onto your back and swing your legs up the wall, keeping your hips close to the wall.

Slide your right foot down the wall, lifting the hips off the floor and bending the knee. Place your left foot over the right knee.

Move the left knee towards the wall and slowly lower the hips until you feel the familiar stretch on the side of your left hip and buttock. Rest with the hips hovering above the floor for at least 25 seconds.

You can experiment with the right heel on and off the wall.
*Change sides and repeat.*

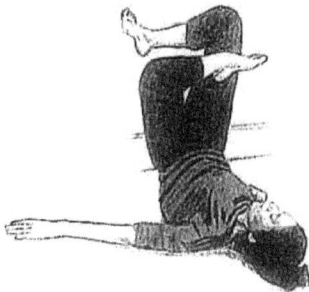

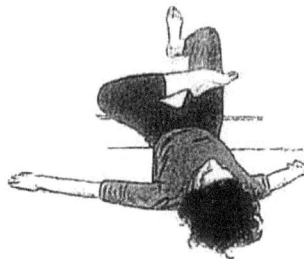

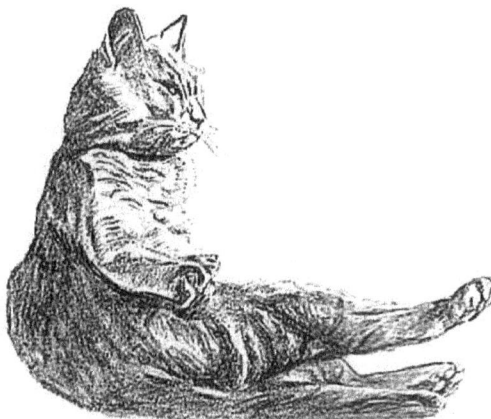

# Introduction to the Groin Stretch Sequences

One of my pupils, who was recovering from prostate cancer, needed stretches for his under-functioning lymph nodes in the groin area. He found the last three stretches, with one hand on a chair, helpful. I developed them while experimenting to find piriformis stretches.

I subsequently came across the first of the four postures, the **Sideways Groin Stretch**, in the book **The Supple Body** by **Sara Black**, see page **48** This motivated me to put together this short sequence.

The original version of **1** is a little different from mine. It says you feel the stretch on the inner thigh of the straight leg and suggests holding the stretch for around 15 seconds. I have expanded the scope of the stretch and increased the duration. Hold for the shorter time if you find it too demanding.

When you are working with the chair, you can either work straight through the three poses and then change sides, or change sides after each one. The intensity of the stretches will evolve as you progress through the sequence. You will feel the stretches more if you pause for about five minutes after doing the sequence, or try different postures, and then return to it.

The **Supine Splits** from the **Giraffe Sequence** in my book **Yoga Sequences Companion**, 2011, is also a good groin stretch.

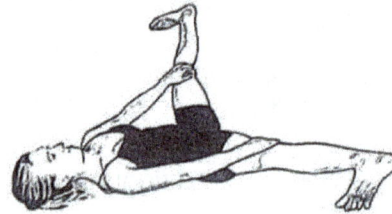

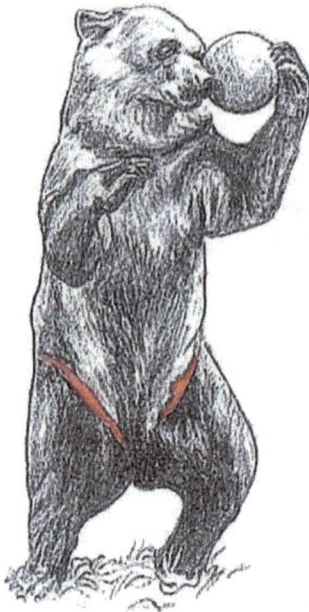

**The groins**

The **groin** is the area in the body where the upper thighs meet the lowest part of the abdomen. Normally, the abdomen and groin are kept separate by a wall of muscle and tissue. The only openings in the wall are small tunnels called the **inguinal** (of the groin) and **femoral** (of the thigh) **canals** that allow nerves, blood vessels and other structures to pass between the two areas.

In the groin, underneath the skin, there are between three and five deep lymph nodes that play a role in the immune system.

**Lymph nodes** are small glands that filter **lymph**, the clear fluid that circulates through the lymphatic system. They become swollen in response to infection and tumours.

The **lymphatic system** is a network of tissues and organs that help rid the body of toxins, waste and other unwanted materials. The **primary function** of the lymphatic system is to transport lymph, the fluid containing infection-fighting white blood cells, throughout the body.

# Groin Stretch Sequence

**1**. Stand with the feet wide apart and at a 45 degree angle. Bend the left knee, move the hips forward a little and lean slightly backwards.

You may not feel the stretch at first and some experimentation may be necessary. A slight shift in the tilt of the hips will move the stretch from the top of the thigh to the groin on either side.

With practise, you may feel it in both groins and thighs. *Hold for at least 20 seconds. Change sides and repeat.*

**Caution**. Stop if there is any discomfort and either persevere with shorter stretches or seek medical advice.

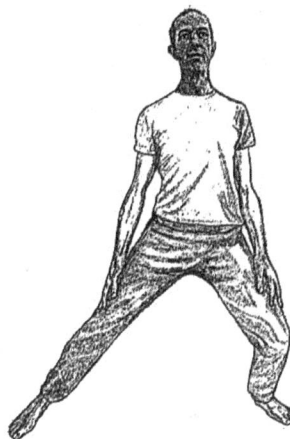

**2**. Stand in front of a secure chair[1] with the feet wide apart. Rotate your right foot to a 90 degree angle and place the right fingertips or hand on the chair behind you.

Look at your left hand as you swing it upwards and back. Move the hips forward and hold the posture as above.

*Either come briefly out of the pose and then continue to* 3, *or change sides and repeat.*

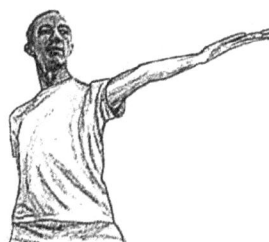

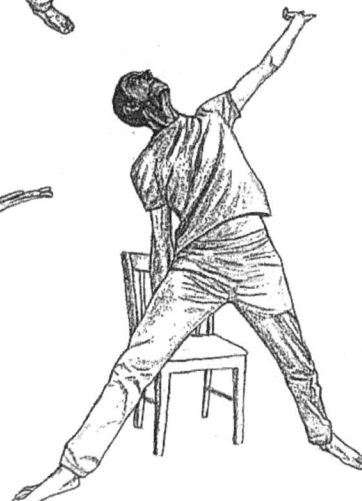

**3**. Bend your right knee and repeat as above.

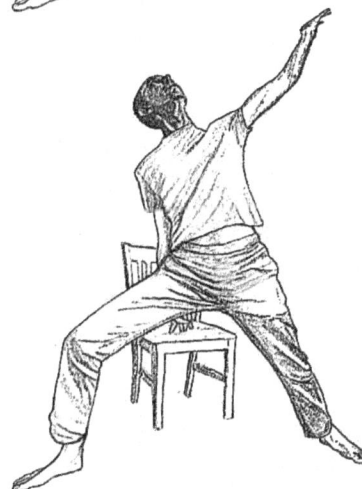

**4**. Go up on your left toes and move into a **Deep Lunge**. Rotate your left heel to a comfortable position and repeat as above.

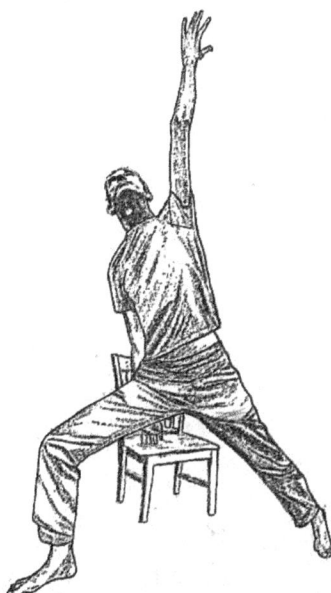

---

**1**. To secure the chair, place the two front legs on the side of your mat, lengthways. This should stop it from slipping and give you sufficient mat space for the postures. If that doesn't seem secure enough, place the back of the chair against a wall, although this is not ideal if you are tall, because it may inhibit your space.

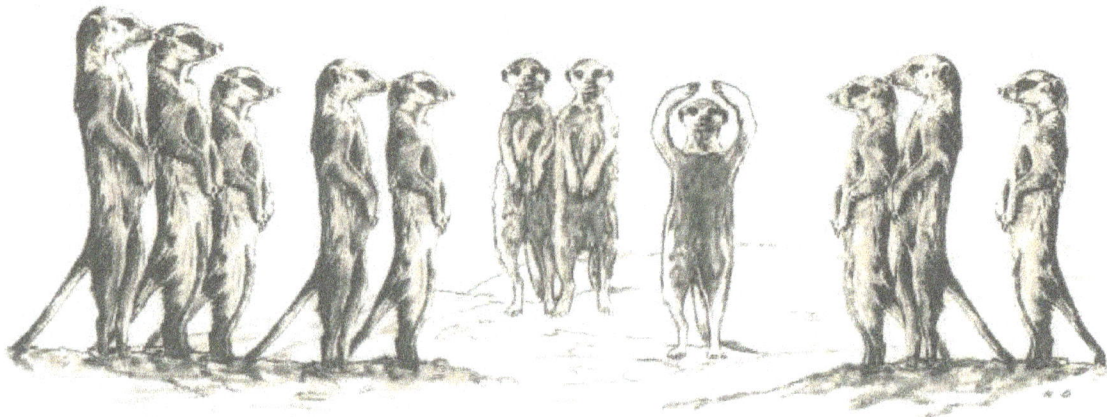

**Meerkat Yoga Class**

# Wave Breathing

Imagine you are standing on a lovely sandy beach, looking out at the waves crashing on the seashore. It is a hot summer's day, and the bright blue sky is reflecting on the sea.

Observe the waves. There is a crest that builds up and curls over into a long trough. Then the energy builds up again into another wave.
Now visualise your breath as a wave and add the mantra:

## Om   Ah   Hum

Crest

A pause while the
energy builds up
again.

Trough

Crest

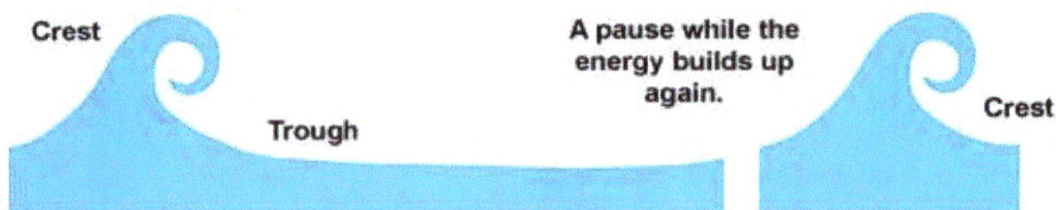

**Inhale, think OM**
**As you go over the top of the inhalation, think AH**
**Subside into a long exhalation, think HUM**
**Pause until you need to inhale again**

After at least eight slow breaths, add the sound of the sea, **Ujjayi** breathing, as described on page **23**. You make the sound of the sea in your throat. You can slowly increase the volume.

# Introduction to the Elbow Grasp Sequence

This is inspired by a sequence in **Yogaflows** by **Mohini Chatlani**[1] It has evolved, and only loosely resembles the original Yoga Flow.

Other influences are from the book, **The Supple Body**, see page 78, in postures **14**, **15** and **18**. **17** and **18** come from a video by **Erin Sampson** of **Five Parks Yoga**. I have added **3** and some variations to the original.

## Additional postures

After **3**, you can make a much bigger circle with your arms as illustrated.

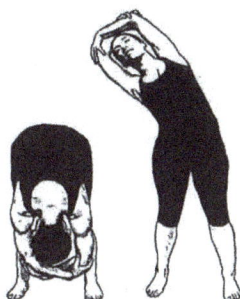

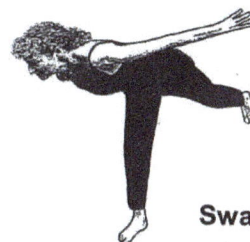

Swallow

You can vary the balancing posture in **12**. You could try the **Half Moon**, **Swallow**, **Tree** or **Balancing Warrior** for example. Try to move from them into **13** without the lifted foot touching the floor.

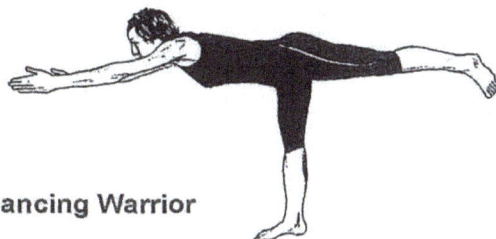

Balancing Warrior

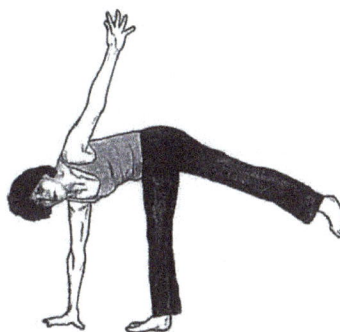

Half Moon

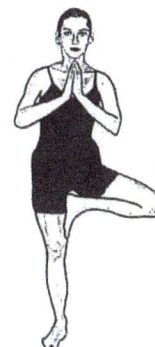

Tree

## Additional notes

I have changed the supporting leg in **12** to accommodate the average practitioner. If you want to make it more demanding, continue lifting the right leg from **12 to 15** and vice versa after you have changed sides to repeat it.

In **3**, I say put your right hand on top when holding your elbows. Continue this instruction each time you hold your elbows. When you repeat the sequence, change sides. Have the left hand on top. This is just a suggestion for appropriate clientele. For some classes this would be **too much detail**.

I developed the **Balancing Postures in Pairs** because it prepares you for **4** and involves the postures I have mentioned above. It is like a prelude to this sequence. I find working in pairs, especially in classes where the same people have been coming for some time, makes people happy. I took the photo of my pupils in **1** and think it proves my point. My pupil is wearing shoes because she has a problem with her feet and ankles.

# Introduction to the Balancing Postures in Pairs

**1** and **2** are from general yogic repertoire. **3** and all the others are from a much longer inspirational sequence in the video **KKY Partner poses for Kids** by **Karma Kids Yoga** of New York. **Shari Vilchez Blatt** is the leading light.

1. Used with kind permission from **Mohini Chatlani** from **Yogaflows**[tm], 2002, published by Ted Smart.
www.heartspaceyoga.com    www.mohinichatlani.com

# Balancing Postures in Pairs

**1.** This is **4** in the **Elbow Grasp Sequence** in pairs. Stand side by side and place the inner arm/hand on the partner's outer shoulder. Catch hold of the outer foot with the outer hand and stretch the leg out to the side. When you have established your balance, move the feet forward and then take them out to the side again. *Changes sides and repeat*.

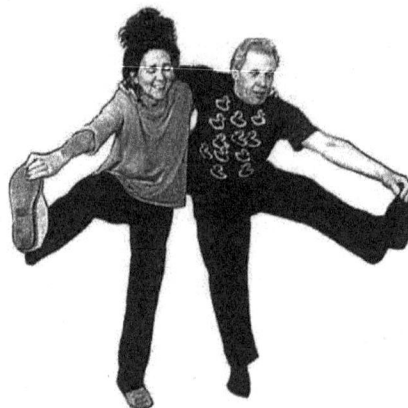

**2. The Tree in pairs**
  You may prefer to position the outer foot before you join the hands. If you can't rest it on the thigh, as illustrated, find an alternative position so that you are standing on one leg.
  Lift the inner hands towards the ceiling and push the palms against each other. Bring the outer hands in front and join these palms together as well.

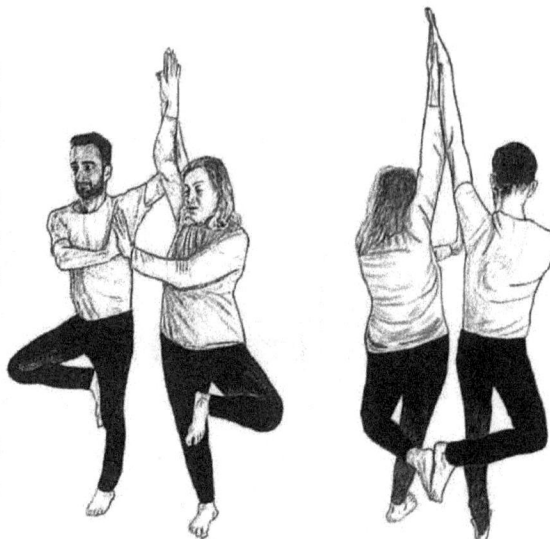

**3.** While keeping the palms together, lower the outside foot and move it behind the inner leg. Connect the souls of the feet together behind. *Change sides and repeat 2 and 3*.

  **From 4** to **6** you are **back to back**. I will call the side facing forwards in the illustration, the **active** side.

**4. Forward facing Warrior (Warrior 2).** Stand back to back with the feet wide apart. One of you will bend the left leg and the other the right leg, on the **active** side. Stretch your arms out to the side and join the hands together. Experiment and find the most comfortable way for you to do this. Turn the **inactive** side feet inwards. *Hold for a few breaths*.

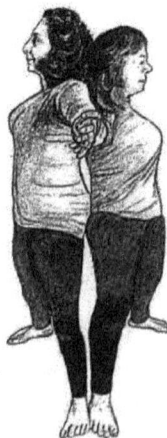

**5. The Triangle in pairs.** Straighten the bent legs. Still holding hands, and keeping the arms straight, lower the hands down towards the feet on the **active** side.

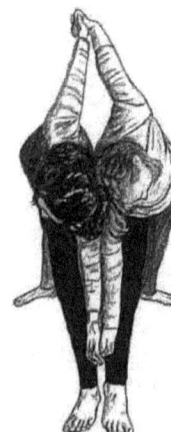

6. **The Half Moon in pairs**. Separate the lower hands. Bend the knees on that side and stretch forwards with your hands, placing the fingertips firmly on the floor, and then straighten the legs once more. While keeping the joined upper hands high, lift the back legs. Let them touch behind if possible. If you feel secure, you might like to bring the front hands together.

*When you are ready, return to 4 and repeat on the other side.*

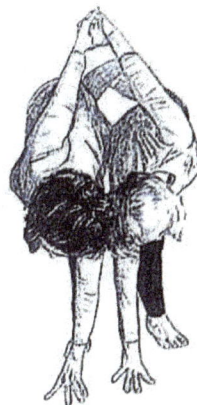

In the **Karma Kids Yoga** video, mentioned in the introduction, the arms are out to the sides rather than forwards as is usual in the **Balancing warrior**. I assume that is because the hands are on the partners shoulders and it is more practical. You could try bringing the hands forwards or swinging them back into the **Swallow**. It may suit some arm/body ratios.

7. Stand side by side again and place the inner hands on your partner's outer shoulder, as in **1**. Lift the outer legs. Hold for as long as you want to.

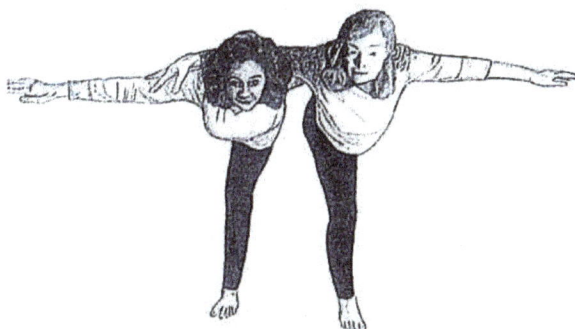

8. When you are ready, lower the outer legs and lift the inner legs. When you are ready, *change sides and repeat 7 and 8.*

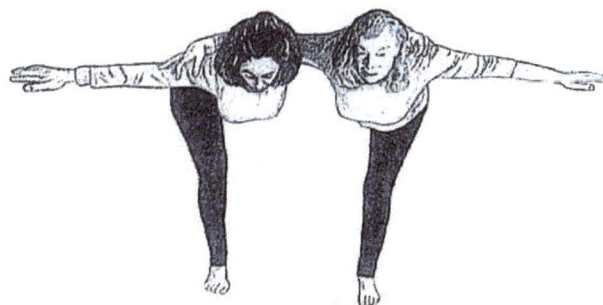

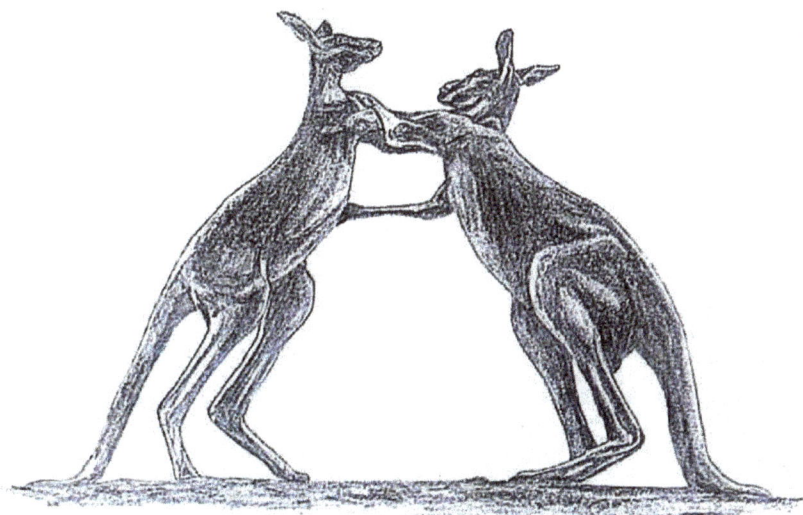

# Elbow Grasp Sequence

1. Stand with the feet together and the hands in **Prayer**.

Venus Lock

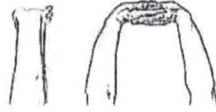

2. INHALE the hands above your head in either **James Bond** mudra (**Ksepana** mudra) or **Venus Lock**. EXHALE over to the right. *Change sides and repeat x2*

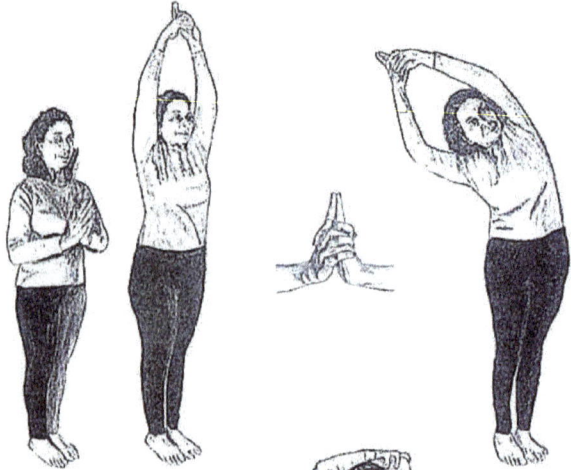

3. **Elbow and Hip Circling**   Catch hold of your elbows with the right hand on top. Circle the elbows, keeping them above your head.   The hips will move in the same direction but on the opposite side of the circle. It takes a bit of practise to get the best results. *Change direction when you are ready*.

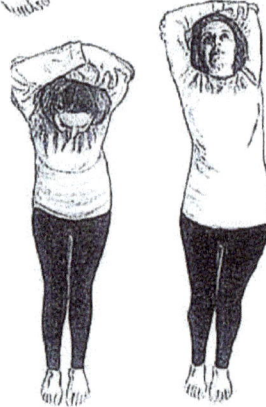

4. Catch hold of your right foot with your right hand and straighten the leg in front.  The left hand can be out to the side or on your hip.  When you have established the balance, you can move the leg out to the side and back.
   If you have difficulty balancing, you can stand with your back against a wall or hold on to the back of a secure chair with your left hand.

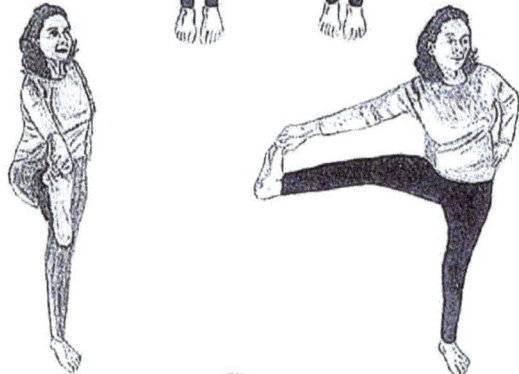

5. Carefully lower the right leg and place it on the floor behind. INHALE as you straighten the legs and turn your right foot to a 45-degree angle. EXHALE as you lower your head to your knee. The hands can be on either side of the foot or on the lower leg. *Hold for a few breaths.*

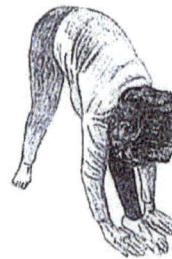

6.   Move your right foot a little further back while bending the left knee.  Go up on your back toes, sinking into a **Deep Lunge**.  You can turn your left heel out to the side a little to help your balance. Slide the right palm down the outside of your left leg until the elbow rests on the knee. Extend your left arm behind you as you twist round to the left. Follow your hand round with your eyes.  Hold for a few breaths.
   If you find this posture too demanding, you can go down on your right knee or rest your left thigh on a chair, as illustrated in 7.

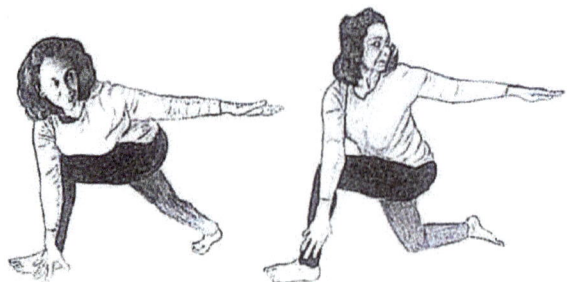

**7.** Twist around the other way, with your left hand on the inside of your left leg and the right arm stretched behind, as in **6**.

If you have bad knees, you can rest your left thigh across a chair, as illustrated. You could also rest on the corner of the chair seat.

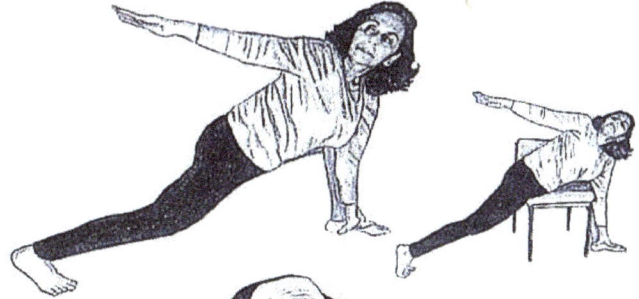

**8.** While holding the twist, catch hold of your elbows with your hands and let the weight of your head and arms lower them towards the floor. You can lower the right heel to the floor. Hold for a few breaths and then *twist round the other way and repeat.*

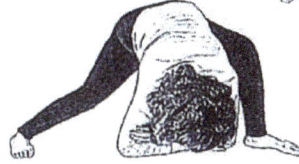

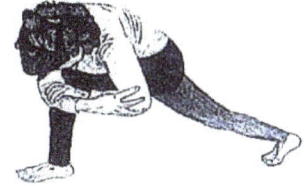

**9.** While twisting round to the left, you can place your right hand on the left shoulder and the left hand on your hip.

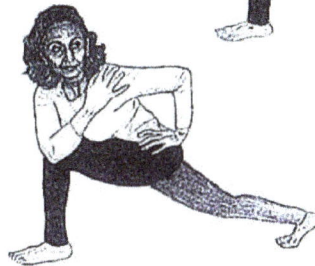

**10.** Lower the hands to the floor in front and then the knees, coming onto all fours. Straighten the right leg out to the side and go up on the right toes.

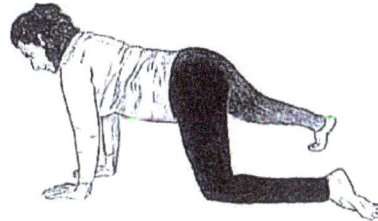

**11.** Swing your right foot around to the left, as far as it will go. Look under your left armpit at your right foot. To increase the stretch, move the left foot and hips to the right. Hold for a few breaths and then swing the leg back to the right, at roughly the same angle. Look under your right armpit at your foot and move the hips a little to the left. **Experiment** with keeping the **arms straight** or **bending the elbows** out to the sides, rotating the fingers inwards as you twist round. *Repeat a few times*.

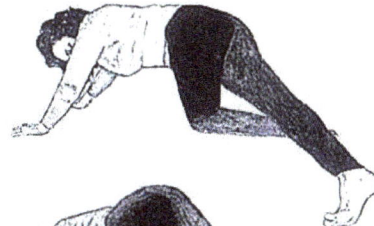

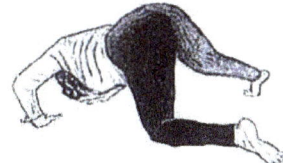

**12.** Bring your right foot close to your right hand and push up into a **Standing Forward Bend**. With your hands on the backs of your legs, or on the ankles, bend the elbows and bring the head towards the knees. Hold for a few breaths.

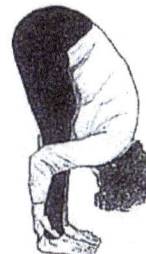

**13.** Prepare to move into the **Standing Splits**. Lunge your head and shoulders forwards as you lift your left leg. Place the right hand on the right calf, bend the elbow and bring the head towards the knee. Lift your left leg as high as you can. Hold for as long as you need to.
**Please see variations for this posture in the introduction.**

**14.** Bend both legs as you bring yourself back up to standing and swing your left foot forwards, without it touching the floor. Hold and breathe, with your right leg bent and the straight left leg hovering in front. Adjust this posture to your level of fitness and flexibility. You could try bending the right leg more and lifting the left leg parallel to the floor.

**15.** Lower the left leg and return to **Standing Forward Bend**. Catch hold of your elbows. Feel the heaviness of the head and the lower spine slowly stretching as you hold and breathe.

**17.** INHALE as you go up on your left toes and EXHALE as you twist round to the right, keeping your head low and resting your arms/wrists on the right leg. INHALE back to the centre and lower your left foot. EXHALE as you go up on your right toes and twist round to the left.
*Repeat as many times as you want to.*

**18.** While still holding your elbows, INHALE as you soften your knees and bring yourself back up to standing. EXHALE as you bend to the right. Hold for a few breaths and then *change sides and repeat*.

**19.** From the central position, open out your arms, lift the chest and lean backwards. INHALE deeply and EXHALE with one of the following: a **Ha Breath**, a deep sigh or one of the mantras of the **Heart Chakra, Yam** or **Om Hreem**.

**20.** *Return to 1 and repeat the sequence*, changing legs in **4** and placing the left hand on top when you catch hold of the elbows.

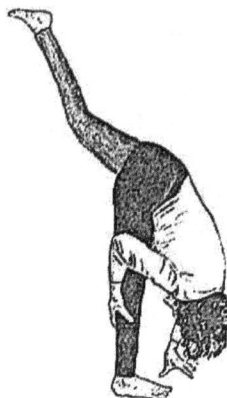

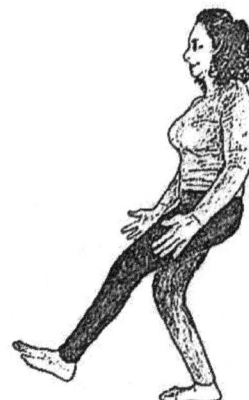

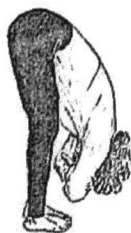

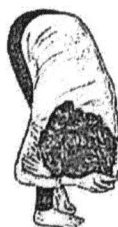

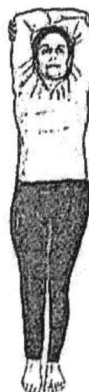

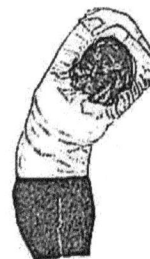

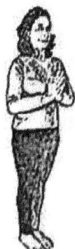

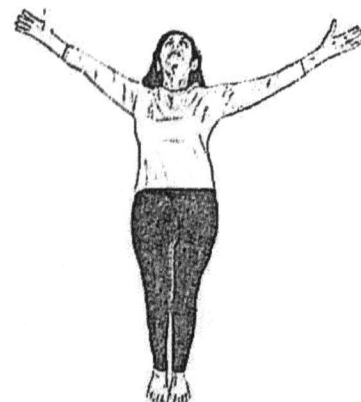

# Sung Meditations

I was taught this Kirtan Kriya by Darryl O'Keeffe at a workshop. Yogi Bhajan, who formed the Kundalini Yoga Movement developed this meditation. I have simplified it to use at the end of my yoga classes. To access the original version type 'Kirtan Kriya, Sa Ta Na Ma' into your seach engine.

**Sa** - the universe, totality
**Ta** - life, creation
**Na** - death, dissolution
**Ma** - rebirth, regeneration

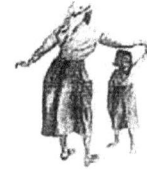

Sing the mantra slowly using this melody at your chosen pitch.

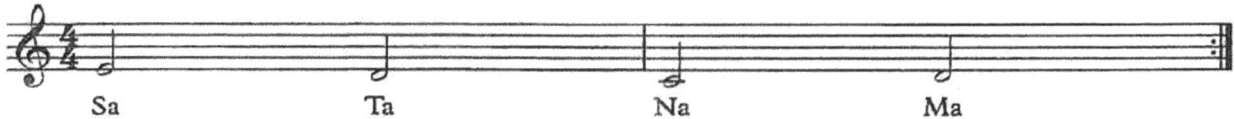

There are four sections. You can pace these according to the time available and your inclination.

1. Sing it about twelve times. Roughly four times very loudly, four times at middle volume and then again softly, gradually reducing the volume until you can hardly hear it.

2. Repeat (intone) the mantra silently for as long as you choose to.

3. Start to sing the mantra again about the same number of times as in 1, but reverse the volumes. Start very softly, move to middle volume and finish very loudly.

4. Repeat the mantra silently again.

Two other mantras suit this format well:
**Om Mani Padme Hum**. This is a Buddhist chant, often translated *Hail the jewel of the lotus flower.*

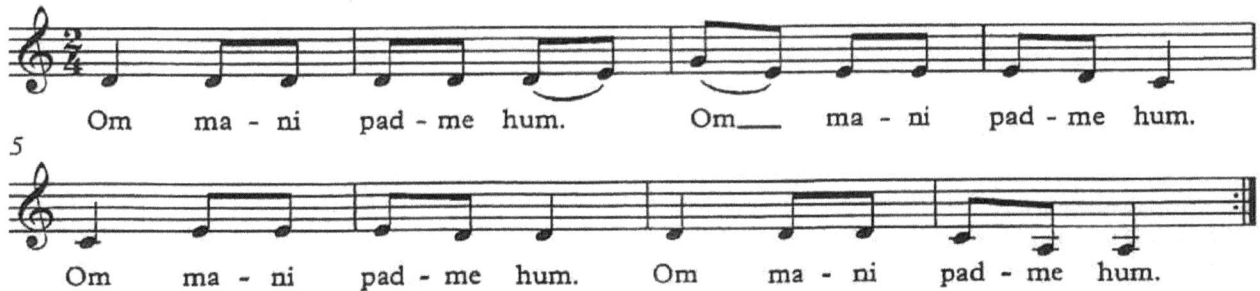

**Shri Ram, Jai Ram, Jai Jai, Ram Om**. Ram is short for Rama. Lord Rama is considered by Hindus to be an incarnation of God. His heroic life story is told in **The Ramayana**.
It translates, *Lord Ram, Hail* or *Victory to Ram.* **Om** is known as the universal sound.

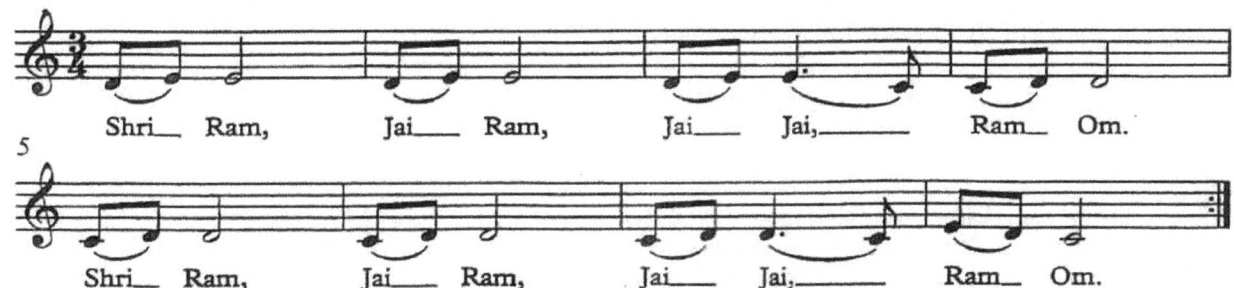

# Triangle Concentration/Meditation

When my meditation was going through a mind-wandering phase, I contemplated using **direction of thought** to control the intruding thoughts. **I started to combine a triangular shape with the breath**. I was surprised at how quickly and completely the mind-chatter disappeared.

When you have mastered the simple method below, you can improvise different triangles and expand the practice.

## Method

Sit in your usual meditation posture. Lift one hand and place two fingers in the middle of the top of the forehead, on the hair line. Place two fingers of the other hand about 3 inches (7cm) above the navel, the **mid-point**. You are touching the top of the triangle and one corner of the base. When you have established these points in your mind, lower the backs of your hands to the thighs and open out the fingers. Feel the energy in the palms of your hands.

Now take your awareness to the tip of your right thumb. That is the other corner of the base of your triangle.

Before you start to INHALE, concentrate on the tip of your **right** thumb. As you INHALE, take your awareness from the thumb to the point at the top of your forehead. EXHALE down to the **mid-point** and then **pause at the end of the exhalation**. During the pause, take your awareness back to the tip of your thumb.

**Repeat this twice more** and, during the third pause, take your awareness to the index (second) finger and repeat the procedure. Work your way through the five fingers of the right hand. That will be 15 breaths.

**To continue**, move on to the **little finger of your left hand** and work your way through the five fingers to the left thumb, another 15 breaths.

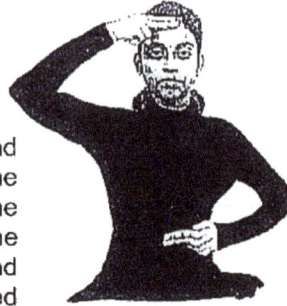

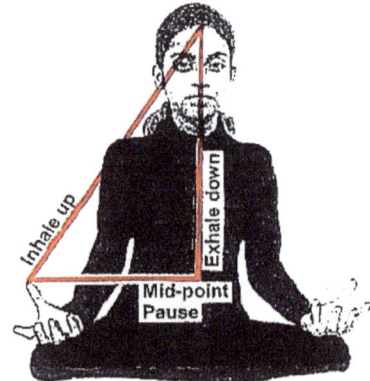

## Additional notes

It **helps if you move each new finger** or pair of fingers **a little** as you connect with them.

Once you have mastered the **concentration during the pauses**, you can appreciate the benefits of this practice. Normally, when you pause after the **inhalation** or **exhalation**, you stop thinking and the mind goes blank. Here, you won't be using words, but feeling and visualising the base of the triangle. Do not start the **inhalation** until you have connected to the top of a finger.

It is difficult to time the pause because that involves using words, but it can be between approximately 3 and 10 seconds, or as long as it takes to bring your awareness to the chosen finger.

When you are familiar with the practice, you can do it lying on your back.

Please see the notes on page 18 about the connection of the hands to the brain.

## Variations

Once you are familiar with this basic practice, you can change the points of the triangle, involve the chakras, start using a mantra or use it as a tool for healing.

**Please note**, it is always best to involve the fingers. The hands contain many acupuncture points and connections to the brain via the nerves, especially in the thumbs. The palms of the hands also emit large amounts of electromagnetic energy. The constant point of your triangle will be the tip of a finger. It doesn't matter how wonky your triangle is.

Here are some variations. You can improvise more of your own.

1.  Use both hands to form the base of the triangle. Start the **inhalation** at the tip of your **left** thumb and take your awareness to a higher point. It could be the one already used or the point between the eyebrows, the **Third Eye** or **Ajna Chakra**. EXHALE down to the **right** thumb and **pause** as you take your awareness back to the tip of the **left** thumb. Continue as before, moving each pair of fingers a little as you move onto them. **This is how I introduce this practice to a class.**

2.  INHALE from the tip of the thumb to the point between the eyebrows. EXHALE to the Acupuncture point **Ren 6**, about 2-3 inches (about 7 cm) below the navel. The Chinese say *the breath starts here*. **Pause** as you take your awareness back to the tip of the same thumb. As before, feel and establish the new points before you begin. You could also change the direction by **inhaling** into **Ren 6**.

3.  INHALE from the thumb to the top of your head, the **Sahasrara Chakra**. EXHALE down to the base of the spine, the **Muladhara Chakra**, and **pause** while you take your awareness back to the tip of the same thumb.

   If you prefer to take your awareness up the spine rather than down it, you can change the direction[1]. Start with your awareness at the tip of the thumb again and INHALE down to the base of the spine. EXHALE up to the top of the head and **pause** as you take your awareness back to the thumb.

4.  **If part of your body is in need of healing,** use that part as one point of the triangle. You will be **exhaling** into the part to be healed. If it is a **shoulder,** for example, you could go from the finger to the point at the top of the forehead, and EXHALE down to the shoulder. **Pause** there, while you take your awareness back to the tip of the finger.

   If it is a **knee** that needs healing, you could INHALE from a finger into the **Heart Centre,** the **Anahata Chakra,** and EXHALE down into the knee.

   As you INHALE, imagine taking in healing energy from the Universe. As you EXHALE, visualise a silvery white light taking that energy to the part of your body that needs to be healed. As you **pause,** feel the healing energy being absorbed into the area while you take your awareness back to the chosen finger.

5.  **To involve a mantra** (see Glossary), combine it with the breath. If it has one syllable, e.g., **Aum (OM),** hear it internally on both the **inhalation** and **exhalation.** If it has two syllables, e.g. **So Hum,** think one on the inhalation and the other on the exhalation. If it has more syllables, find a way to coordinate it with the breath.

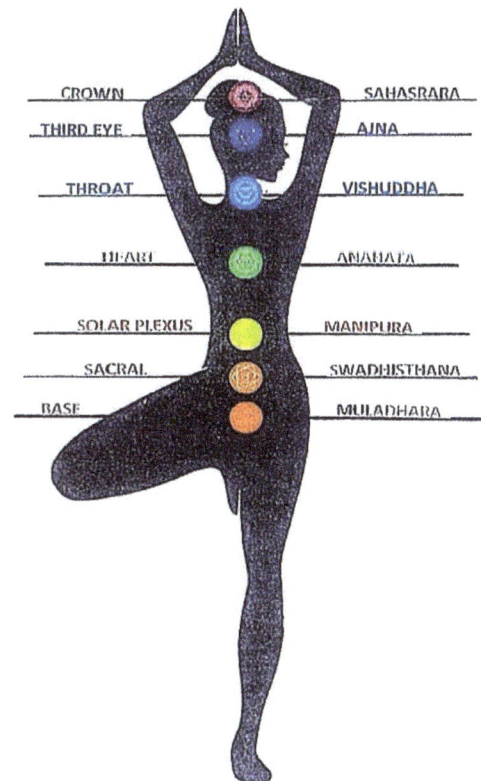

| | |
|---|---|
| CROWN | SAHASRARA |
| THIRD EYE | AJNA |
| THROAT | VISHUDDHA |
| HEART | ANAHATA |
| SOLAR PLEXUS | MANIPURA |
| SACRAL | SWADHISTHANA |
| BASE | MULADHARA |

**The positions of the Chakras**

1.  Visualising energy moving **up the spine** has implications for raising the Kundalini. People who have experimented with recreational drugs should proceed with caution when practising this variation. They are more susceptible to random rising of the Kundalini. If they, or anybody else, feel stirrings or odd sensations at the base of the spine, they should stop immediately, unless they purposely want to raise their Kundalini. Be warned that it can have positive and negative consequences.

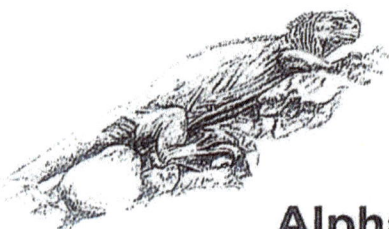

**Iguana**
A herbivorous lizard.

**Umbrellabird**
from the rainforests of Central
and South America

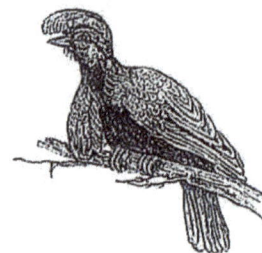

# Alphabet Meditation

My brother George told me about this meditation. It is very simple and keeps the mind 'on track' very effectively.

## Method

**Choose a category** that has lots of different names. Here are three obvious ones:

1. **Living creatures**, i.e., animals, birds, reptiles, insects and fish.

INHALE and think **A**.

EXHALE slowly and think of a creature's name that starts with **A**, e.g., Antelope.

INHALE again and think **B**.

EXHALE and think of a creature's name that starts with **B**, e.g., Butterfly.

Carry on all the way up the alphabet. That will be **26** breaths. If you get stuck and can't think of a corresponding creature, don't take any extra breaths; just go on to the next letter. I have given a few ideas for letters you are likely to get stuck on.

2. **People's names**. These can be from any language.

INHALE and think **A**.

EXHALE slowly and think of a person's name that starts with **A**, e.g., Anne.

INHALE and think **B**.

EXHALE and think of somebody's name that starts with **B**, e.g., Benedict.

It will take about 6 minutes to work your way through the alphabet. **For a longer meditation or variation** go back to **A** and start all over again. This time, use longer **exhalations** and think of more names per letter. For example, if you were on **D**, it could be **dog, donkey, dolphin** or **dragon fly**. For people's names it could be **David, Daniel, Daphne** and **Diana**. On **K** it could be **kangaroo, kingfisher** or **komodo** (dragon). For people's names it could be **Kate, Kevin, Keith** or **Kayli**.

For a meditation/relaxation at the end of a class, I like to go through the alphabet once using one name per letter and then repeat it using multiple names.

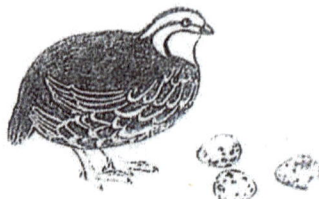

**Quail**
Small bird of the partridge family

**Xoloitzcuintli** (Xolo dog)
A hairless Mexian dog

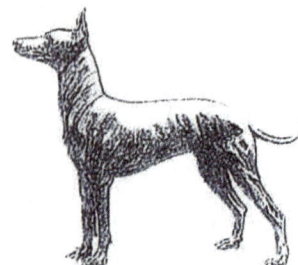

**Another variation** is to think of girl's names the first time you go up the alphabet and boy's names the second time, or vice versa. Here are some names for letters you may have difficulty with:

**Girls**

Olive, Queeny, Ursula, Una, Undine, Xabrina, Xena, Yvonne, Yvette, Yulai, Zoe, Zena, Zarah.

**Boys**

Oliver, Quin, Quincy, Quentin, Unvin, Uli, Xavier, Xander, Xylon, Xain, Yevgeny, Yehudi, Yavin, and Zachary.

3. **Names of continents, countries, towns and places.**
Use the same method, **inhaling** and thinking the alphabet letter and **exhaling** slowly and thinking the name of a place on planet earth.

Here are some you may struggle with: Queensland, Quebec and Xenia (in Ohio), Xai Xai (in Mozambique) and Xanthi ( in Greece).

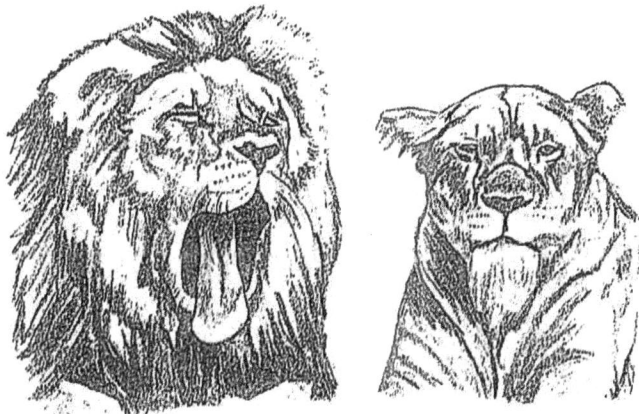

# Vedanta, the Vedas and the Upanishads

*The self is everywhere. Whoever sees all beings in the Self, and the Self in all beings, hates none. For if one sees oneness everywhere, how can there be delusion or grief?*
The **Isha Upanishad** (probably between 1,000 and 500 BC).

**Vedanta** is often called **the End of the Vedas**, *anta* means **conclusion** in Sanskrit.

The **Vedas** are a large body of religious texts originating in ancient India, 1,500-700 BC (dates vary).They deal with meditation, mantras, philosophy, spiritual knowledge, benedictions, rituals, ceremonies and sacrifices. **Veda** means *knowledge*.

The **Upanishads** played an important role in the development of spiritual ideas. Vedanta was an integral part of their message. They initiated the transition from Vedic ritualism to a broader perspective. There are 108. The first 12, the most well known, were most probably written before 500BC. The remaining 95 were written between about 100BC and 1400CE. They were translated and brought to the West in the early 19th century.

# Loving Kindness Salutation[1] for the end of a Yoga Class

This is another idea gleaned from Tasha's[2] classes.  She says she learnt it from one of her former teachers, Amir Jaan.

   After the final relaxation, if you were on your back, roll over onto your right-hand side and come to sitting.  Bring the hands into **Prayer** at the **Heart Centre**.  Become aware of the **energy** in the **palms of your hands** and allow your **body** to become a **sacred temple**.
   **The teacher** says the words that go with the hand positions.  The class can join in if they want to.

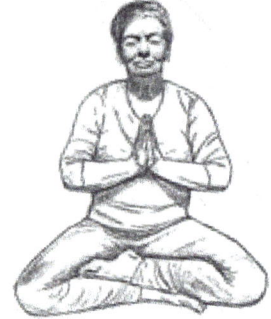

Place the hands on the **Crown of the head**.

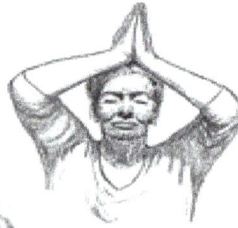

**Peace for all**

Lower them to the **Third Eye**

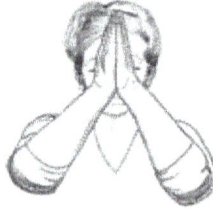

**Light for all**

Lower them to the **Throat Centre**.

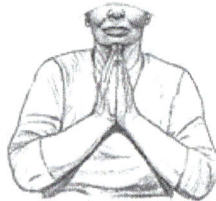

**Truth for all**

Lower them to the **Heart Centre**.

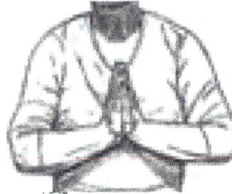

**Love for all**

Lower them to the **Solar Plexus**.

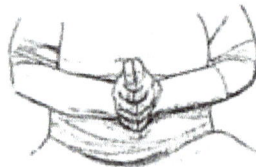

**Compassion for all**

**Safety and Security for all**

Place your hands on the floor in front.

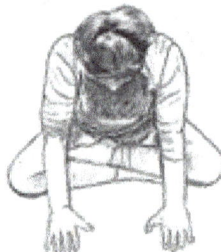

1.  My name for it.  I am not aware of another name.
2.  See page  41

# Introduction to Loving Kindness Visualisation

**Loving Kindness meditation** has a long history. It is called **Maitri** in Sanskrit[1] and **Metta** in Pali[2]. It is usually translated to mean **benevolence, loving kindness, friendliness, good will and active interest in others**. *Brahma-loka* was an ancient Hindu *Highest Heavenly Realm* practice based on the **four virtues** of **loving-kindness, compassion, emphatic joy** and **equanimity.** These concepts are found in Buddhism, the early Upanishads[3] of Hinduism and also in the early Sutras of Jainism[4], where they were called **Maître** or **Metta**.

The Buddha never claimed that the *four immeasurables* and related **Metta** meditation were his unique idea, but **Loving Kindness** meditation is usually known as **Metta** in yogic circles today.

This passage is taken from the Buddhist text, **Karaniya Metta Sutta[5]**.

*May all beings be happy and secure; may they be happy-minded.*

*Whatever living beings there are - feeble or strong, long, stout or medium, short, small or large, seen or unseen (ghosts, gods and hell-beings), those dwelling far or near, those who are born and those who await rebirth -- may all beings, without exception, be happy-minded.*

*Let none deceive another nor despise any person whatever in any place: in anger or ill will let them not wish any suffering to each other.*

*Just as a mother would protect her only child at risk of her own life, even so, let him cultivate a boundless heart towards all beings.*

*Let his thoughts of boundless loving kindness pervade the whole world: above, below and across, without obstruction, without any hatred, without any enmity...*

Here is another example of Buddhist thinking by Lama Thubten Zopa Rinpoche:

*Compassion is the best healer. The most powerful healing comes from developing compassion for all living beings.*

## Visualisation Notes

**The paragraph in green** can be replaced during the Christmas period with the alternative paragraphs, also in green, on the opposite page. **Pauses at the end of paragraphs** are necessary.

**The source of this particular Loving Kindness visualisation**
I have used this visualisation at Christmas for many years but I can't remember where the original idea came from. I suspect that the basic concept came from a meditation workshop a long time ago and I have added my own ideas.

**Caution** I would not use this visualisation if I was teaching individuals who were displaced or leading lonely, dysfunctional existences. It might emphasise their isolation and loneliness.

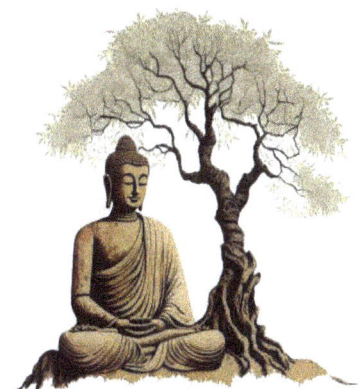

Image courtesy of pngtree.com/so/buddha'

1. Please refer to the **Glossary** for a definition of **Sanskrit**.
2. **Pali** is a Middle Indo-Aryan liturgical language (language of ritual and works of a spiritual nature) of the Indian subcontinent. It is the language of the **Pali Canon** and the sacred language of **Theravada Buddhism**.
3. **The Upanishads** are a series of sacred Hindu treatises written in Sanskrit between 800 and 200 BC. There are twelve principle Upanishads. They are philosophical in nature.
4. **Jainism** is an ancient Indian religion usually noted for its support of **non-harming** and **vegetarianism**.
5. This is a shortened passage from the **Wikipedia** site, **Metta Meditation**. The translation is by Peter Harvey.

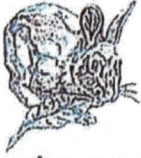

# Loving Kindness Visualisation

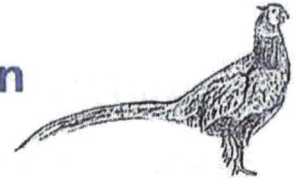

**Imagine you are sitting at the top of a hill** overlooking rolling countryside. There are a few trees behind you and clumps of trees dotted across the landscape, but the countryside is mostly grassland. Sheep are scattered over the hillside and way down at the bottom of the hill there is a field with a few cows and horses in it. There is a village in the valley with a church to one side.

**There isn't a cloud in the bright blue sky** and the afternoon sun is high above. All we can hear is the sound of birds singing and the occasional sound of sheep *baa-ing* in the distance.

**We are going to imagine** that sitting next to us, at he top of the hill, are **our nearest and dearest;** close friends and family. Some of them may need our forgiveness and compassion. We are going to wish them all well and send them our loving kindness.

**A little further down the hillside** are the people we **see on a regular basis in our lives.** They could be people we work with, those who serve us in shops or the bank, or those we meet when we do our favourite things. We will probably never go to their homes or know details about their lives, but we care about them and want them to be happy. Extend your emotional warmth and empathy to them and send them your loving kindness.

**Further down the hillside** are the people we **see and learn about in the media,** in newspapers and on television, et cetera. We will probably never meet them or communicate with them, but they are still part of our lives. We hear about their trials and tribulations and their happy times and we feel for them as fellow human beings. If we don't like some of them, we can think about their backgrounds and try to understand how it influenced them. Try to develop compassion for all living creatures. From your heart, send them all your loving kindness.

**At the bottom of the hill** are the many people who live around us. They are **pulling strings in the background,** growing food, policing our cities, organising, caring for people, et cetera. They are part of our lives; we know they are there but we never notice them. Send them your loving kindness.

**Way down in the valley,** stretching for miles and miles and following the rivers down to the lowland, are all those billions and billions of people who share this planet with us. We will never get to see or know about them. We hear about them in large groups, never individually, but we still care about them. We would still like them to be happy and free of suffering. Feel warmth and compassion for them in your heart and send them your loving kindness.

**From the top of the hill,** look at all the people on the hillside and in the valley at the same time, and feel warmth in your heart for them all.

**Find yourself back inside your body** and bring your awareness to the breath.

## Alternative paragraphs for a Christmas Visualisation

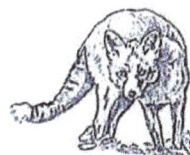

**We are going to imagine** that sitting next to us, at the top of the hill, are our nearest and dearest; close friends and family. They are the ones you might give Christmas presents to or maybe spend Christmas day with. Hold them in your heart, wish them well and send them your loving kindness.

**Close by on the hillside** are the people you send Christmas cards or seasonal greetings to. Some of them you see regularly and others only now and then. Some you haven't seen for years, but they are still important to you. You are sending the message that you haven't forgotten them and you still care about them. Send them all your loving kindness.

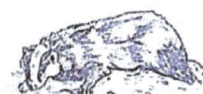

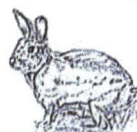

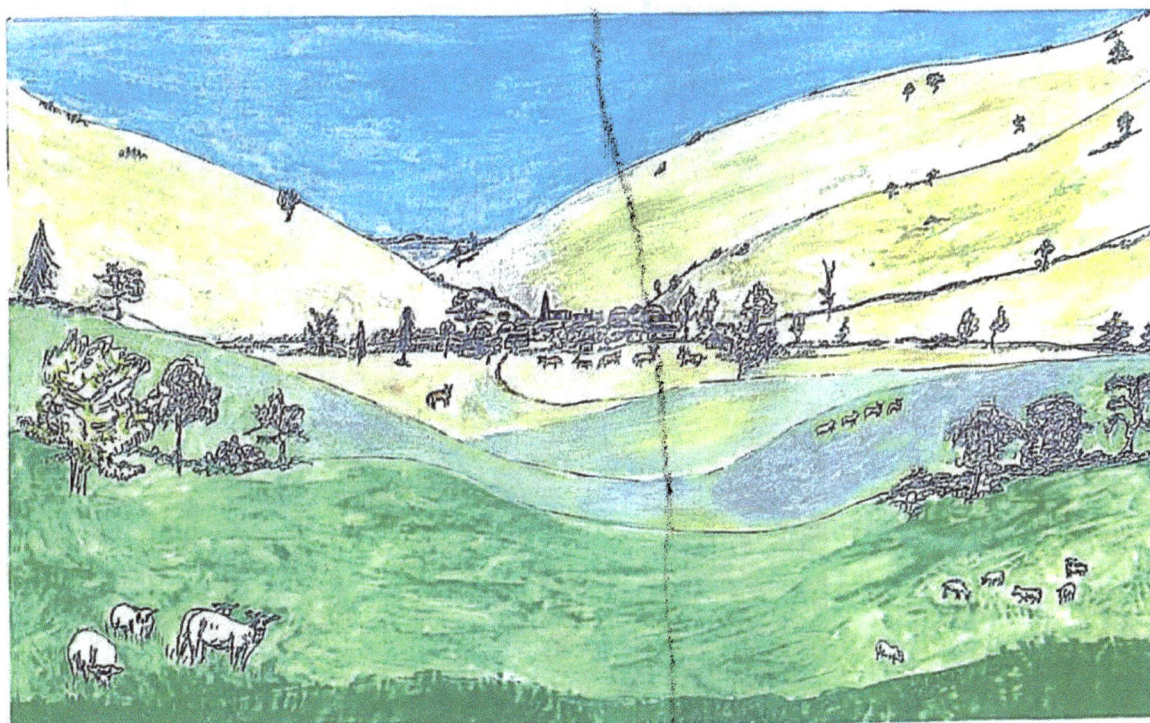

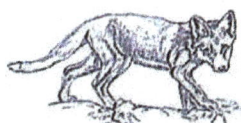

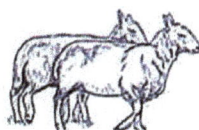

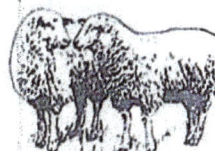

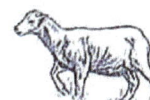

I looked for a photo of a landscape suitable for this visualisation but couldn't find one, so I made a quick sketch of the scene I saw in my mind. I then added a watery wash of colour.

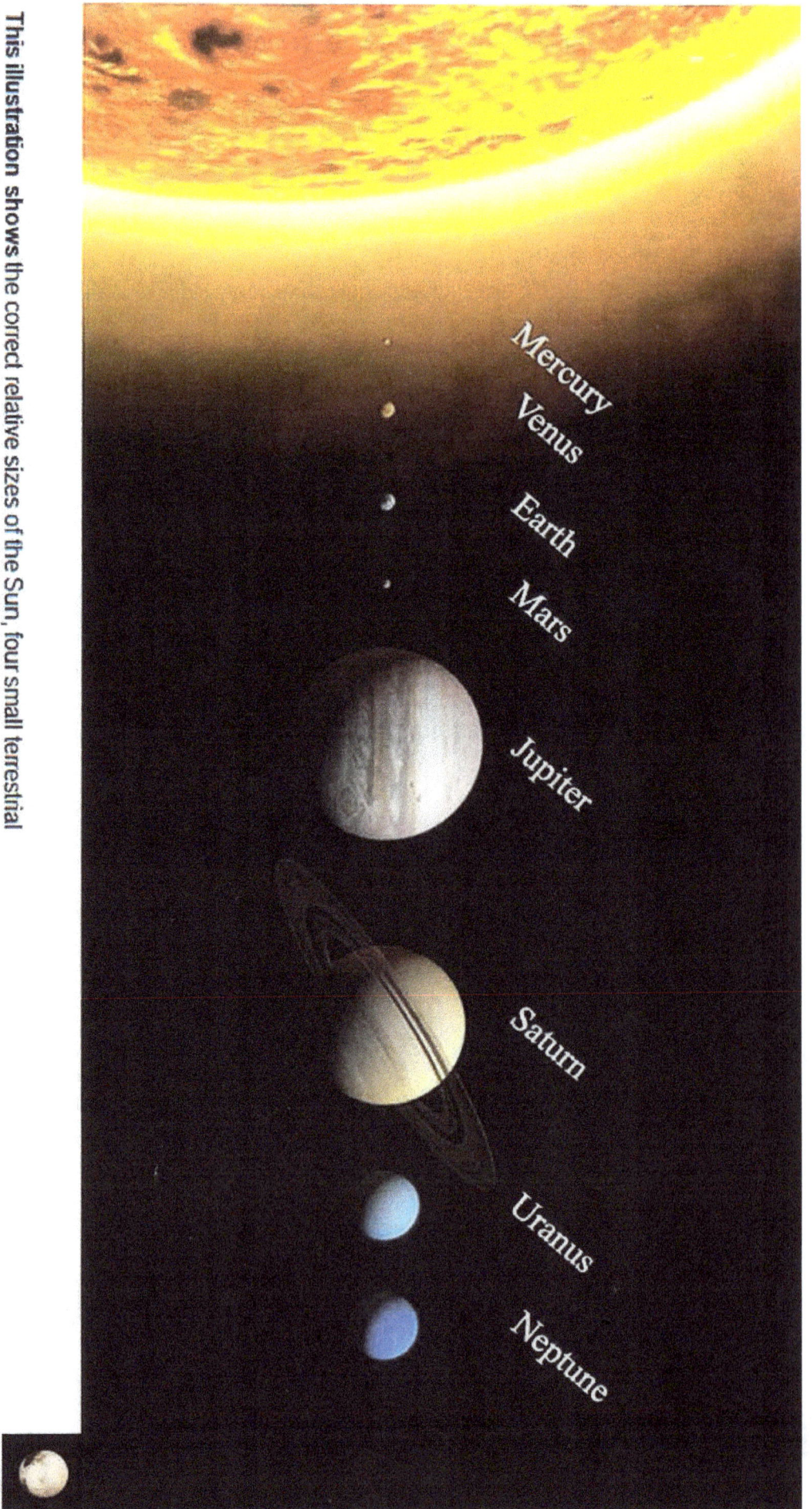

**This illustration shows** the correct relative sizes of the Sun, four small terrestrial planets and the four giant planets. The distances apart are not correct. (Illustration by courtesy of Wikipedia)

**Observe the size of the Sun**. It is about 1,000 times bigger than Jupiter.

**This is Pluto**. It is not in scale with the planets above.

# Introduction to Journey into the Universe Visualisation

When I first started teaching yoga in 1998, I came across an undated tape cassette by **Jean Taylor**, a therapist and meditation teacher, called *Release, Experience guided Relaxation. Journey around the World and into the Universe*. It was my introduction to the art and potential of creative visualisation

Since then I have taken my pupils on many journeys out of our solar system at the end of classes. Eventually, I made up my own version of the visualisation.

When it came to writing my script down, complications arose. My knowledge of astronomy is limited but I have tried to be accurate with the facts. This has proved difficult because scientists often change their minds about planets and the universe as knowledge expands. For example, when I started writing it up I didn't think Pluto was considered a planet anymore. Then a friend enlightened me. It was downgraded to a Dwarf Planet in 2006 by the International Astronomical Union but some eminent astrophysicists don't agree with this assessment and still consider it a planet. Its diameter is two thirds that of our moon and it would not show up on the illustration on the opposite page. I have included a photo of it for those who would like to include it in their journey but have decided not to visit it on our journey as it is quite long enough already. Similarly, I have had to change the age of Jupiter's red spot from *millions* of years to *hundreds* of years. Maybe we don't really know how old it is.

Knowing a few details about the planets helps you to identify with them. Most diagrams of our Solar System show the planets in a straight line. This can show their relative sizes but, as you can see in the diagram accompanying the illustration of the Milky Way below, they are scattered all over the solar system. I have tried to minimise the practical complications while visiting the planets.

Teachers need not keep rigidly to my script. They can retain as much detail as is appropriate for their individual pupils. Some of the text will need to be changed to adapt to your circumstances. The words in red will need to reflect the place where you are on planet Earth. If you are in Scotland, or another country, you will see your own landscape as you leave and return to the planet. I live in the south of England, hence the places I have mentioned. I have used *you* and *our* but you could also use *we*.

**It is necessary to pause** after each new idea/paragraph with a **very dramatic pause after the blue paragraph**. This is the climax of the visualisation. The imagined involvement with our Universe could have different levels of interpretation and reflection. You may want to add your own spiritual interpretation here.

To conclude, I have found Professor Brian Cox's television series about our Solar System deeply inspiring. It was his mind-blowing programme about the planet Jupiter that influenced my choice of background for the cover of this book.

Information about the CD and free sound tracks of this visualisation can be found on page 104.

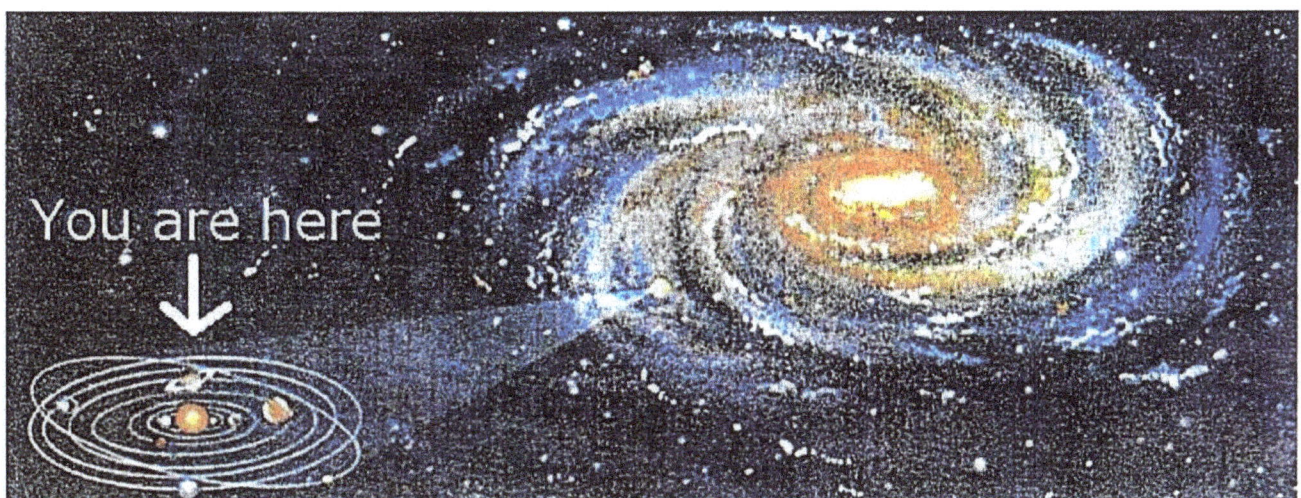

Original Image from: blendspace.com

# Journey into the Universe Visualisation

**Imagine you are standing on the road outside this building** (improvise around your present situation). It is a lovely sunny afternoon. The birds are singing. You look up at the bright blue sky and see the white fluffy clouds floating by.

**Let your awareness expand** and find yourself floating up towards the sky. When you look down, you see the rooftops, roads and trees below becoming smaller and smaller as you float up higher and higher.

**Now you can see the towns and villages** for miles in each direction (give details). The roads connecting them look like twisting grey threads across the landscape. The motorways and railway lines are wider and straighter.

**You float up higher and higher** until you can see hundreds of miles in each direction. Now you can see London and Bristol on opposite sides and right across the English Channel to France and all the way up to the north of England.

**By the time you leave the Earth's atmosphere** you can see all the way down to Italy and northern Africa, across the North Sea and Atlantic Ocean and up past Scotland. Now you can see the circular curve of our planet and the white clouds wrapping around it.

**You are going to take a journey out of the solar system** so you turn away from the sun and drift towards the red planet, Mars.

**Looking back at Planet Earth** from a distance, you will see clearly the part that is facing the sun and, on the dark side, the lights from the towns and cities creating patterns across the land masses.

**You look up at our moon.** It has just risen above the other side of the planet. The side facing the sun is shining brightly. You can just make out the craters and shapes on the surface and the feint outline of the rest of the moon. You can see Venus and Mercury far away in the distance. They are closer to the sun and look much smaller than planet Earth.

**On you go towards Mars.** It shines like a rusty red globe in the blackness of space. As you get closer, you see a few dark areas and lines, some higher landmarks shining in a lighter bronze colour, and gullies that are dry riverbeds. It used to have lots of water.

**You move past it** and notice rocks of different sizes and shapes floating between Mars and Jupiter. You pass between them. This is the Asteroid Belt.

**Jupiter is the largest planet** in our solar system. It is the first of the two gas planets. 1,300 planet Earths could fit inside this majestic giant. You can see bands of colour encircling the planet. These are swirling clouds of browns and greys and blues and white. The texture looks like a cross between a slab of marble and a Monet painting. There is a red ball in one of the brown bands. This is a gas storm that has been raging for hundreds of years. It is the same size as Planet Earth. We see some of its four large moons orbiting around it.

**On you go, moving further away** from the sun into the outer solar system. The next three planets are also giants. They are much further apart from each other than the four, small terrestrial planets. The other gas planet, Saturn, and its rings, are shades of yellow and brown with darker bands in the rings. The rings are very large, beautiful and mysterious. There are at least nine moons but you don't notice them much as you pass by because Saturn and its rings capture your attention.

**The last two giant planets,** Uranus and Neptune, are ice planets. They are so far away from us that we just see a round glow in the distance from them. Uranus is a very light turquoise blue and Neptune is a darker blue (like a blue hyacinth).

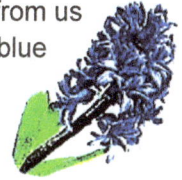

**As we leave our solar system**, we have to pass through lots of frozen objects. They are different sizes and shapes. Pluto is one of the largest. It is now considered a Dwarf Planet because it is only two thirds the size of the Earth's moon. This is the Kuiper belt. It is twenty times wider than the Asteroid Belt

**On and on we go**, further and further out into space. Our solar system is situated on an outer curve of our galaxy's spiral. You look across our galaxy. It is a spiralling swirl of billions of bright shining stars. It gets very dense in the middle where there is a light-coloured glow that looks a bit like milk. This is probably why it is called the Milky Way. Our solar system is just a tiny part of the swirling mass before you.

**You look around into deep space** and see lots of other galaxies in every direction, shining in the blackness of our Universe. **This is the Cosmic Dance of Creation**. Let your awareness take you further and further out into the cosmos as you drink in the beauty and energy of deep space.

**Eventually, it is time to return to Planet Earth**. You find yourself near Neptune, but first you have to cross the Kuiper Belt, all those different shaped boulders of ice that circle around the edge of our solar system. You pass slowly through them towards the blue planet Neptune. As you move past it, the intense blue with narrow streaks of white, seems to go on forever.

**Now you can see the distant glow of Uranus**. On and on you go until Neptune fades into a little blue ball floating in the blackness. Uranus is a vast glowing mass of white and pale greeny-blue ice. The softness of the gentle colours is soothing.

**You pass by Uranus** and see Saturn far away to the left. Because it is so large and the background of space is so black, you can still see the rings and yellowy-brownish colours clearly. It looks just as awe-inspiring from afar.

**The next one, nearest to the sun,** is majestic Jupiter. You cannot help being drawn to its energy, splendour and beauty. As you get closer, you notice the swirling bands of coloured textures on the surface. These are all fierce storms raging in its layers of gas.

**From Jupiter, you can see planet Earth** on your right and the strange rocky shapes of the Asteroid Belt flying in between. We see the part of our planet that is facing towards the sun. You might see a familiar continent peeping out from under the clouds. On the dark side, the lights from our towns and cities remind us that we are not far from home. You travel through the Asteroid Belt and see Mars in the distance to your left. The warm, rusty red colour looks welcoming, which is just as well, because astronauts from planet Earth are planning to go there soon.

**Now you prepare to return to our home planet**. As you approach, its outer curve gets wider and wider and the clouds expand in every direction. You find yourself moving through the outer layers of the atmosphere and into the clouds. You pass through them and slowly start to recognise the landscape below. There's the south of England - there's London - that's the M4. On you go, getting closer and closer to your home town. Fortunately, the sun is still shining brightly and the birds are singing to welcome you home. You notice the familiar trees, rooftops and buildings as you finally land on the road, in exactly the same place where you started your journey.

**Now find yourself back inside your body.** Feel the parts of your body that are making contact with the floor. Slowly bring your awareness to your breath and slow down your exhalations. Every time you exhale, feel your body sinking further and further into the floor. Feel yourself getting heavier and heavier .... and heavier. *Continue for as long as you want to and finish up with a prayer of gratitude for your existence on Planet Earth and the wonder of Creation* (if appropriate).

# The Glossary

**Advaita Vedanta.** The **creator** and the **created** are considered one and the same. Matter is energy vibrating at different frequencies. This echoes Einstein's equation, $E=MC^2$, meaning **energy = matter**. The different dimensions and spiritual landscapes are energy functioning in different ways. In some philosophies and religions the **creator** and **created** are two separate entities.

**Ashram.** Usually a secluded residence of a spiritual community with teachers, and often based around a particular Guru.

**Bhagavad Gita.** This is a dialogue between Lord Krishna and Arjuna, from about 2,000BC. It was transmitted orally for many generations and finally narrated by Vyasa in about 550BC.

**Hatha Yoga.** This is one of the four paths of yoga as described by Lord Krishna in the Bhagavad Gita. Hatha Yoga develops the full potential of the body and mind through systematic practices. These include Asana (posture work to keep the body fit and connected to the brain), Pranayama to utilise the vast energy potential in the human being, and meditation to utilize the full potential of the mind.

**Hatha Yoga Pradipika.** This is a classic Sanskrit manual, written by Swami Svatmarama in about 15th century AD. It is derived from old Sanskrit texts and his own experiences. It advises the aspiring yogi on how to develop an intense spiritual practice.

**Heart Centre.** The area associated with love and compassion in the middle of the chest.

**Kundalini.** This is usually depicted as a powerful energy coiled like a snake or serpent at the base of the spine. Awakening the Kundalini can be spontaneous or controlled. There are many different experiences associated with it, e.g., in Tantric Yoga it can have sexual connotations. In the Hatha Yoga Pradipika it is a disciplined controlled awakening brought about through many hours of Pranayama.

**Mantra.** This is a verbal vibration, or resonance, that has a beneficial effect on the body and mind. It can be spoken, sung or thought. It can be one or more syllables, a phrase, a sentence or many sentences. The Hail Mary in the Roman Catholic Church is a long mantra but there are longer ones in the Jewish canticles. A mantra is repeated many times and used as a point of concentration to steady the mind. People can make up their own mantras, and sometimes a particular word takes over a person's mind and it appears that a mantra has been given to them.

**Maya.** This is the rope that binds man to the illusory world. It is the power which makes form appear real.

**Pranayama.** *Prana* means **life force** and *ayama* means **control** or **mastering**.
It involves many different methods of breathing. When these are combined with other techniques, such as the **Bandhas**, our energy potential can be developed.

**Pratyahara.** Withdrawing the five senses away from the outside world and directing them inwards.

**Samskaras.** Deep mental impressions produced by past experiences. They can be dormant impressions from our past lives.

**Sanskrit.** This was the language of the ancient civilisation which developed on the banks of the Indus River in what is now Pakistan. We find the earliest evidence of yoga there.

**Throat Centre.** This is the Vishuddha Chakra in the throat. It acts as a bridge between the higher and lower intelligence in the body. What is felt there will be a reflection of the relationship between the abdomen, heart and brain in the head.

**Vedanta.** It means the *end of the Vedas*. *Ante* means **conclusion**. There are different school of Vedanta but the most influential is **Advaita Vedanta**, as taught by **Adi Shankara** in about the 8th century (dates vary). *Advaita* means **not two**.

**Vedas.** A large body of religious Indian texts dating from about 1,500 to 700 BC. *Veda* means **knowledge**. They touch on most spiritual and social topics, including rituals and sacrifices.

**Upanishads.** A large body of Indian spiritual texts. The first twelve, the most well known, were most probably written before 500 BC. Vedanta is an integral part of their message.

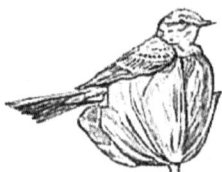

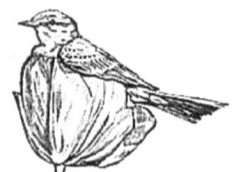

# Yoga Without Boundaries CD

**1. Coherent Breathing** with Piano Accompaniment by Oliver Williams.
Breathing five times a minute, for relaxation and stabilising the Nervous System.
**2. Coherent Breathing** with Piano Accompaniment by Griff Johnson.
As above.
**3. Journey into the Universe Visualisation**
Narrated by Vani Devi, with percussion backing by Aziz Kazi.
**4. Journey into the Universe Visualisation**
As above, with piano track by Griff Johnson.

It can be used in conjunction with the book, **Yoga Without Boundaries by Vani Devi,** or by itself, **for individual or group relaxation and breath awareness. All necessary pages from the book come with the CD.**

# Breathing tracks, 1 and 2

**You need to understand the following facts about the Coherent Breath before you listen to these tracks.**

**Stephen Elliott** is credited with the development and articulation of the **Coherent Breathing** method. **The New Science of Breath,** 2005, by **Stephen Elliott** and **Dee Edmonson, RN**, is published by Coherence Publishing. I learnt about it in 2015 at a workshop given by **Dr. Richard Brown** and **Dr. Patricia Gerbarg** in London. Both are Psychiatrists in America.

**The Coherent Breath** is defined as slow, gentle breathing through the nose at a ratio of **5 breaths per minute**. It involves **inhaling** for **6 seconds** and **exhaling** for **6 seconds**. This rate of breathing accesses the **mid-point** between the **Sympathetic** (which speeds up) and **Parasympathetic** (which slows down) branches of the **Nervous System**. It is like being in neutral gear when driving a car.

Dr. Brown says this breathing ratio activates the **Vagus Nerve**. This is the nerve associated with the **Parasympathetic Nervous System**. However, although the **6-6 ratio** accesses the **mid-point** mentioned above in people of average height, it is different for **children** and **very tall** people.
For children it is breathing **10** times a minute, with a **3/3 ratio**. They can still use the breathing tracks, halving the counts of six. For tall people it is only slightly slower (4.5 breaths per minute) so they should still benefit from using the **6/6** ratio.
<u>Caution</u>   Those with breathing problems, e.g. COPD, should proceed with great caution and stop as soon as there is any discomfort.

# Visualisation Tracks, 3 and 4

You will appreciate the visualisation more if you study the enclosed illustrations of our Solar System and Galaxy before you start listening to it.

**Additional notes.** You will notice variations in the text between the two tracks. Track 3 is the original one. After receiving feedback from pupils, I changed a few things. Also, it was necessary to change the age of Jupiter's red spot from *millions* to *hundreds* of years after reading conflicting estimates. Maybe we don't know how old it is.

# Information about the Artists

### Oliver Williams

Oliver studied Piano at the Royal Academy of Music in the 70s, where he won several prizes. Since then he has led a varied musical life, giving solo recitals, accompanying, teaching, arranging and, in recent years, leading a function band. In 2019 he joined a Flanders and Swann tribute act, as Swann!

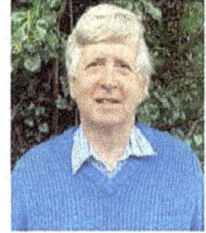

### Griff Johnson

Griff studied Piano at the London Trinity College of Music in the 1980s. Since then he has worked as a composer, arranger, improviser, transposition and keyboard technician, etc., in many different situations. These include working in the theatre in many successful West End shows, touring nationally and internationally with Musical Theatre productions and famous artists, including Shirley Bassey, The Supremes and Rick Astley.

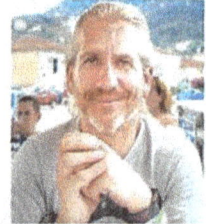

### Aziz Kazi

Aziz is from Karachi, Pakistan. He is a multi-instrumentalist. In this recording he is playing a hang drum, tuned to 432 Hz which is a natural healing frequency. It was recorded at A for Aleph (Artists Residency and Recording Studios) in Karachi.

I sent him a track of me narrating the visualisation after a pupil, who knew him when he lived in the UK, sent me a very impressive video of him playing different instruments.

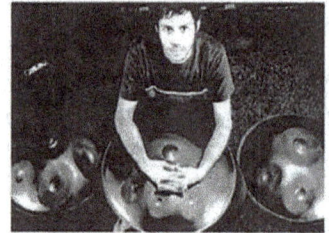

### Vani Devi

Vani (Kate Oppel) studied Singing, Guitar and Drama at the Guildhall School of Music and Drama, London, in the 1960s. She took a Sivananda Yoga Teachers Training course in 1998 and has subsequently taught yoga and written books about it. 'Yoga without Boundaries' is her sixth yoga book. She wrote the script for the visualisation.

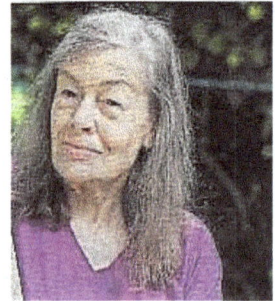

The CD can be purchased from www.koolkatpublications.co.uk for £6.50 plus £2 P & P. The free sound tracks can be downloaded from the same website.

9 780952 478164